Too Young

Too Young to Feel Old

The Arthritis Doctor's 28-Day Formula for Pain-Free Living

Richard Blau, M.D., F.A.C.R.

WITH

E. A. Tremblay

Da Capo
LIFE
LONG

A Member of the Perseus Books Group

Da Capo Press is a member of the Perseus Books Group

Text design by BackStory Design
Set in 11.75 point Bulmer MT

A CIP record for this book is available from the Library of Congress.
ISBN-10: 0-7382-1115-X
ISBN-13: 978-0-7382-1115-2

First printing, October 2007
Visit us on the World Wide Web at http://www.perseusbooks.com

Da Capo Press books are available at special discounts for bulk purchases in the United States by corporations, institutions, and other organizations. For more information, please contact the Special Markets Department at the Perseus Books Group, 2300 Chestnut Street, Suite 200, Philadelphia, Pa. 19103, or call (800) 255-1514, or e-mail special.markets@perseusbooks.com.

Note: The information in this book is true and complete to the best of our knowledge. This book is intended only as an informative guide for those wishing to know more about health issues. In no way is this book intended to replace, countermand, or conflict with the advice given to you by your own physician. The ultimate decision concerning care should be made between you and your doctor. We strongly recommend you follow his or her advice. Information in this book is general and is offered with no guarantees on the part of the authors of Da Capo Press. The authors and publisher disclaim all liability in connection with the use of this book. The names and identifying details of people associated with events described in this book have been changed. Any similarity to actual persons is coincidental.

To Candi, Brandon and Margaux.
Their love and support has been my inspiration not only for this book,
but for my work and my life as well.

CONTENTS

INTRODUCTION

I have been treating arthritis, in all of its many forms, for more than twenty years. During that time, I have seen people of all ages—kids and adolescents as well as younger, middle-aged, and older adults battle with pain and stiffness that intrudes on their lives every moment of every day.

As physicians, we learn many things in medical school, but the most important lesson is to listen to our patients. Mine have taught me that it makes no difference whether you're a teenager, a mother of three, a graying businessman, or an active retiree; we all want to be able to perform at our peak, to go through our life feeling well. Arthritis keeps us from doing that. Unlike most other illnesses, it's *always* reminding us of its presence through the constant pain it causes.

That pain can wear you down. It can make you feel older than you are. When it hurts every time you take a step, every time you brush your hair, every time you move, there is no such thing as performing at your peak or going through life feeling well. In fact, you go through life feeling downright old.

Most of my patients are a feisty bunch. They don't want to sit there and passively hand over their care to a doctor. They want to know what they can do to help themselves, and they haven't been shy about sharing their own remedies with me (some of which actually work). In response, I have taken what I believe to be the best research, science, recipes, exercises, and supplements—along with my patients' best input—and put it into a program that can relieve the pain, stiffness, and swelling of arthritis in a few short weeks.

It is my hope that you will find this book both an easy read and a source for factual information about arthritis for either you or a loved one. In it, I have tried to combine the best of traditional medicine and the best of complementary medicine into an integrated plan of attack. It is time for you to regain your life, renew your vitality, and feel youthful again. After all, no matter what your age, you are too young to feel old.

CHAPTER 1

Arthritis:
You Don't Have to Live with It

IF YOU BELIEVE that joint pain is a natural and inevitable consequence of aging, you're certainly not alone. Most people do. The idea is that our parts wear out just like the moving parts of a car's engine, and there is nothing we can do about it. Sounds logical. Seems reasonable. And it would be if we were made of metal and plastic. Luckily for us, we're made of tougher stuff.

Unlike a car, the human body is composed of material designed to repair and maintain itself. It mends bones, heals wounds, kills germs, gets rid of poisons, and performs millions of other complex biological processes every day in order to stay healthy, whether we're young or old. That doesn't mean that our parts never wear out, but with a little tender, loving care from its owner, a body can get through a lifetime feeling good, strong, flexible, and young.

The fact is that there's nothing predestined about joint pain. It's no more natural or inevitable than diabetes or cancer. It isn't necessarily associated with age, and it often has nothing to do with the "natural wearing out" of the body's tissue. The pain comes from a common disease, so let's call it what it is: arthritis.

Arthritis has many causes and appears in more than one hundred forms, the two most common of which are rheumatoid and osteoarthritis. Whatever the variety, however, from the everyday to the most exotic, they

1

all share one characteristic in common: joint inflammation. It's that inflammation, not wear and tear, that is the hallmark of the disease and the main cause of its symptoms: pain, swelling, and stiffness.

Like many diseases, you're better off dealing with arthritis in its earliest stages, but unfortunately, that rarely happens. Why? Because as mentioned above, people believe joint pain is an inevitable, natural consequence of aging, so when they first begin to feel it, they don't take it seriously. Here's a typical story.

Wendy's Rude Awakening

Wendy was a 51-year-old office manager who gave piano lessons to school children in the evenings to earn extra income for her family. With a garden to tend on the weekends and a hyperactive Border Collie to care for—not to mention a husband, a teenage daughter still living at home, and three grandchildren who frequently came for visits—slowing down never seemed an option for her. She depended on her body to be up, running, and in perfect condition every morning at 6 a.m. And so it was . . . until a morning arrived when it didn't seem quite as perfect as usual.

On that day, she awoke to strange sensations in her hands, especially her fingers. When she tried to move them, she felt a sharp twinge, almost like a bad sting, followed by a cold, achy stiffness. Several times she balled her fingers into fists, as if tightening and un-tightening them would work out the kinks, but that didn't help much.

She felt an even sharper jolt as she turned the valve handles in the shower stall, and a new ache in her hand below her thumb made her drop her bar of soap. She tried to remember if she had demonstrated any particularly demanding passages for one of her piano students the previous evening. It was the only explanation that made sense—except that she had touched the keyboard only twice to play a simple scale. So if not the piano, then what? What had she done to herself? Then the unthinkable occurred to her: *Maybe I didn't do anything to myself. Maybe I'm just getting old.*

She shook her head. The day had to come sooner or later. Well, there was no time to sit and stew about it. It was just another change she would have to get used to—like graying hair and "age spots."

By the time she left the house for work, her discomfort had begun to subside, and by mid-morning, it had gone away completely. She didn't think about it again until the following morning . . . when it came back. In fact, from that time forward, it made an appearance nearly every day.

Eventually, it became part of her morning routine. She tried to shrug it off, although sometimes the pain was severe enough to make brushing her teeth or lifting a cup of coffee a little more difficult. It also lasted longer into the day now, and she found that occasionally she had to give her fingers a rest from the computer keyboard. She began using an over-the-counter pain reliever to take the edge off. That helped a little, but the aching and stiffness remained persistent.

More Than a Feeling

Wendy finally began to take her pain more seriously when she noticed some tenderness and swelling in the joints just below her fingertips, which doctors call the *distal interphalangeal* or DIP joints. For many of us, seeing is believing, and believing means worrying. It's much harder to stay in denial when the evidence is right in front of you, twenty-four hours a day, seven days a week. Something was wrong with her hands, and she feared she might have to stop giving piano lessons. She had already reached a point where she was explaining far more than demonstrating to her students. It was time to see a doctor.

For Wendy, that meant her family physician, whom she'd been with as a patient for more than twenty years. (At this point in the progression of their disease, people will generally come to see me, a joint specialist, only if a friend or relative—most likely a current patient—passes my name along. Otherwise, their regular doctor is their natural choice.)

Predictably, Wendy's doctor didn't take her condition much more seriously than she did. His advice: "You've got a little arthritis. Take some Aleve, and you'll be fine."

Of course, that's what she had already been doing for months—and now her stomach was beginning to pay the price with burning, cramping, and even nausea. So she figured she would just have to live with the discomfort in her hands. That might have been the end of the story had the pain remained only in her hands, but eventually, she developed tenderness in her knees as well. This time she was tempted to blame it on kneeling in the garden, but just in case it might be something more serious, she returned to her doctor. He referred her to me.

Assessing the Challenge

The first thing I do when I see a patient like Wendy is give her a thorough medical evaluation. Among other things, that meant a general physical exam. As a rheumatologist, I understand that systemic diseases can make their first appearance as joint pain. So we needed to know if she had any medical conditions—such as thyroid disease or diabetes—that might cause a secondary form of arthritis.

It also meant her answering a series of questions designed to determine how much her problem had forced limitations on the way she lived her day-to-day life—what she could and could not do, and to what degree her pain interfered with normal activities.

I asked her about difficulty getting out of a chair, walking up steps, brushing her teeth, combing her hair, cutting food with a knife, writing with a pen or pencil . . . about 30 different activities in all. The test was very subjective, of course, but that's exactly what I wanted. I see thousands of patients a year. To my eye, someone like Wendy might seem pretty average in terms of her discomfort, but my opinion doesn't matter.

MAKING LIFE A LITTLE EASIER

A roll of Wonderliner by Griptex shelf and drawer liner is invaluable in the kitchen. It is non-slip and washable. Cut squares and use them under mixing bowls to hold them in place. They are also very useful in helping to grasp jar lids for better grip and easier opening. You can find this product in the kitchen section of most department stores, online, or at specialty kitchen stores.

Wendy was the one who had to cope with her limitations, not me, and if she perceived her pain as being severe, then that was the standard we would work from.

After all, this is a real quality of life issue. People with heart pain may become aware of it only when they exert themselves, but people with arthritis feel it every single time they move. Ordinary activities—ones you probably take for granted such as wiping yourself when you go to the bathroom—become a chore.

Wendy rated her discomfort during each activity on a scale from one to ten, ten being the worst. (By the way, my patients do a new pain assessment at every visit so that I can follow their progress over the days, weeks, months, and years.) She rated her pain at an average of six, but felt it sometimes flew up to eight.

That's a relatively high level, but she seemed to be doing okay with it. She was able to function, go to work every day, and give piano lessons in the evening. Still, there was no reason for her to continue living with all that discomfort if she didn't have to—and she really didn't have to. I offered her three options, any one of which would have brought her relief:

- Physical and Occupational therapy consisting of exercise and heat treatment of the affected areas.
- Medication that could be taken orally for her hands, and in the case of her knees, an injection with a substance that acts like an artificial cartilage.

- Alternative therapy consisting of supplements (especially omega–3 fatty acids), a special anti-inflammatory diet, and an exercise routine that might not only relieve pain but dramatically reduce inflammation as well.

Wendy's Choice

Physical therapy is a good option for some folks, but for those, like Wendy, who have extremely busy lives, taking several hours out of their day two or three times a week is simply too difficult. Medications can work miracles, but sometimes they can also have side effects—occasionally very powerful ones, such as Wendy's stomach problems. Alternative or "complementary" treatment, on the other hand, is inexpensive, requires a minimal time commitment, and for people with mild to moderate disease, can be just as effective as the other two approaches and sometimes even more so. Not surprisingly, this was the option that Wendy chose.

My recommendations for her started with diet. As I mentioned above, all forms of arthritis are diseases that cause tissue inflammation in the joints. Inflammation is an important weapon in your immune system's arsenal against wounds, infections, and other insults it has to fight off or heal every day. It's what causes you to have a fever when you're battling against destructive bacteria, viruses, or parasites in your system. It's also what kickstarts the skin around that cut in your finger to begin knitting together.

Excessive or inappropriate inflammation, however, often proves too much of a good thing. We've recently learned, for example, that inflammation in the arteries can lead to the buildup of circulation-stopping plaque, which in turn can cause a heart attack or stroke. Recent research also strongly suggests that cancer can be the outcome of the body's inflammatory processes. We know for certain that the pain and swelling of arthritis is the result of uncontrolled inflammation.

The Food Connection

Many of the foods we eat support the body's inflammatory reactions. When we have destructive inflammation, however, supporting it with diet may not be such a good idea. So for Wendy, we recommended that she start cutting back her consumption of certain items, including fried foods, most processed baked goods, and anything made with corn oil, safflower oil, butter, margarine, or shortening. These foods are rich in omega-6 and omega-9 fatty acids—fats that the body converts into substances called arachidonic acids, which in turn become pro-inflammatory compounds (actually hormones) called prostaglandins.

The typical American diet generally contains too many of these foods and too few of those containing anti-inflammatory compounds such as omega-3 fatty acids. So I also recommended to Wendy that she increase her consumption of omega-3 foods, which include deep water fish (wild salmon, tuna, cod, mackerel), whole grains, certain fruits, vegetables, nuts, and other anti-inflammatory spices and condiments, including ginger, turmeric, and garlic. I also suggested that in place of corn oil she should cook with more healthful oils such as walnut, olive, canola, or macadamia nut (which you can even use for frying). Flaxseed oil is a great choice for salads.

Because a diet that is well balanced in omega-3s and omega-6s also tends to be low in simple carbohydrates and unhealthful fats, it would also help her lose weight, which in turn would take some of the pressure off of her knee joints.

The Dos and Don'ts of Supplements

To give Wendy's omega-3 intake an even bigger boost, I recommended that she take some fish oil every day. Fish oil comes in either capsule or liquid form. The capsules can be pretty large and difficult to swallow, so most of my patients have switched to taking a couple of teaspoons of the

MAKING LIFE A LITTLE EASIER

Closing a button or pulling up a zipper can sometimes be difficult if you have hand problems. Fortunately, they make a small helpful aid to give you extra leverage in performing these two tasks. For about ten dollars you can make getting dressed so much easier. Your local pharmacy or surgical supply company can order one for you, or you can go online to www.Sammonpreston.com to see all of the aids to assist in daily living.

liquid form. For those of you who may have grown up being force-fed cod liver oil, which has one of the foulest tastes known to man, that's not the fish oil I'm talking about. Pharmaceutical grade fish oil generally comes from salmon, not cod's liver, and it is so super-purified that it has much less of the fishy taste or smell of the old-fashioned home remedy your mother gave you. In fact, several brands have added flavors like lemon, orange, and ginger to the oil, which make it quite pleasant to take.

I also told Wendy she had the option of taking flaxseed oil or flaxseed meal as a supplement. Flaxseed also contains anti-inflammatory fatty acids.

As many of my patients do, Wendy asked about using a combination of glucosamine sulfate and chondroitin sulfate to treat her disease. These two substances have gained quite a bit of media attention because of their supposed ability to heal arthritis by growing new cartilage.

Actually, the body produces both substances naturally. Glucosamine is a sugar that commonly appears in connective tissue such as cartilage. Chondroitin is a carbohydrate that helps cartilage retain water. Unfortunately, there is no evidence whatsoever to show that either one, when taken orally in supplement form, can regenerate damaged tissue in a joint. In fact, it makes sense they *wouldn't* work. Otherwise, they would somehow have to 'know' how to find their way to specific locations in the body, where they could be used to repair damaged tissue.

There is some evidence that they can relieve pain, although that too is controversial. In a study called GAIT (The Glucosamine/Chondroitin

Arthritis Intervention Trial), funded by the National Institutes of Health, the supplements did barely better than a placebo at reducing mild to moderate osteoarthritic knee pain. However, there was some evidence that they could be of greater use in treating severe arthritic pain. Other studies have shown either the combination or glucosamine alone to be about as effective as acetaminophen (Tylenol) at reducing pain. My own experience with patients has led me to agree with these latter studies.

Treating for Pain

So then, Wendy asked if she should use them instead of over-the-counter (OTC) pain medications. Frankly, I couldn't see why she would want to. While it's true that OTC drugs like Tylenol and Aleve can have side effects when used improperly, so can glucosamine/chondroitin. Some recent studies, for example, have suggested that they may reduce the effectiveness of a class of drugs called statins, which are used to lower cholesterol. They may also block blood thinners like coumadin.

Bottom line: If you're not taking other drugs that may interact with glucosamine/chondroitin, I don't recommend against their use, but I can't see that they have any advantage over OTC medications, and they're far more expensive. By the way, for people who follow kosher dietary laws, these supplements are out of bounds. Often they're made from byproducts of the meatpacking industry—to be more specific, the tracheas of pigs and cows.

In the end, the goal was to get Wendy off all pain medications—or at least to the lowest dose possible. Pain is caused by two factors. First, there's mechanical pain, which simply comes from two bones rubbing together when the cartilage between them is too worn down to provide a cushion. Second, and far more importantly, pain is a byproduct of the inflammatory process, which manufactures a class of proteins, called cytokines, that cause pain. If the anti-inflammatory supplements and diets relieve pain by reducing inflammation, the need for pain medications is often reduced or even eliminated.

THE MANY FACES OF ARTHRITIS

Gout: It has been called the disease of kings, and with good reason: Alexander the Great, Charlemagne, and Henry VIII all suffered with it. To be fair, so did some famous folks in democratic countries—Ben Franklin and Thomas Jefferson among them. Left untreated, gout is an extremely painful, disabling form of chronic arthritis that often starts as an excruciating pain in the big toe, but can also affect other joints in the feet and ankles, as well as the wrists. Its cause lies in a build-up of uric acid in the blood. The acid forms tiny crystals that settle into joints, where their sharp edges can cause irreversible damage. You're at higher risk for gout if you're obese and/or have diabetes, high cholesterol, high triglycerides, or high blood pressure. Fortunately, modern medicine offers very effective medications to treat the disease, but dietary changes are most important of all. Start by avoiding red meat and seafood, as these are very high in nitrogen-containing compounds called *purines,* which the human liver converts into uric acid. Alcohol intake should be limited, but does not need to be eliminated.

In addition to dietary changes and supplements, I recommended an exercise program for Wendy. These included range-of-motion and stretching exercises to help maintain her flexibility, strength exercises with light weights to help fortify the muscles that supported her joints, and cardiovascular exercises to help her keep her weight under control and her circulatory system in good condition.

Good Results

As patients get better, I'm looking for an eighty percent improvement. Wendy, like many patients, said she would be happy with just fifty percent. How do we judge? We're looking at two main indicators: how patients say they feel generally and the results of their pain scale evaluations. If I can get them down to a five or three, I'm happy. But most get down to a two, one, or like Wendy eventually did, a zero. And it doesn't take long. If there's no damage showing on the x-ray, we'll probably begin to see that kind of improvement in a couple of weeks. At most, it shouldn't take more than a month.

Unfortunately, Wendy waited nearly a year to get help and suffered a great deal when she really didn't have to. She's not alone. The majority of undiagnosed arthritis patients put up with a lot of unnecessary pain. As time goes on, they rearrange their lives and limit their activities more and more in an effort to avoid discomfort. As a doctor, it saddens me to see this happen, because the solution is so simple, safe, effective, and fast— and people just aren't aware of it. That's the bad news.

The good news is that at this very moment, you're educating yourself. With the program presented in this book, not only will you achieve significant relief from your arthritis symptoms, but you'll improve overall health and lose unwanted weight as well.

Taking the First Step

Just as no two people are exactly the same, even identical twins, neither are any two cases of arthritis. That's why the Arthritis Doctor's Program provides a flexible approach to arthritis management, which you'll tailor to fit your personal needs.

The first step in designing your program is to find out where you are right now in terms of your discomfort. As I mentioned above, patients who come to the Arthritis Institute of Long Island answer a fairly long questionnaire to assess their pain at every visit. That gives a very detailed picture of their condition, which is medically very helpful. But for self-assessment, a much simpler set of questions will tell you what you need to know.

Take a look at the Arthritis Doctor's Questionnaire (ADQ) below and answer each with *never, sometimes, often,* or *always*:

- Do you have morning stiffness?
- Do you have joint pain?

- Do you have muscle pain?
- Do you have difficulty lifting a cup?
- Do you have difficulty cutting your food?
- Do you have difficulty getting out of a chair?
- Do you have difficulty walking on flat ground?
- Do you have difficulty walking up steps?

Now score your answers as follows:

Never = 0 points
Sometimes = 1 point
Often = 2 points
Always = 3 points

If your ADQ score is less than 8, you may have mild or early stage arthritis. In the *Arthritis Doctor's Program,* you'll handle your symptoms with supplements and exercise. Diet is optional, although I would still recommend it, given its other health benefits.

For a score between 8 and 16, you most likely have moderate or mid-stage arthritis. Your program will consist of supplements, exercise, and an anti-inflammatory diet.

For a score of greater than 16, you'll begin a program of supplements, exercise, an anti-inflammatory diet, and an exercise routine, but I would also strongly recommend that you seek medical attention. You may have advanced arthritis, or your arthritis may be a symptom of some other medical condition.

Now you have a point of reference. Let's take a look at what's actually going on in your joints.

CHAPTER 2

The Face of the Enemy

ARTHRITIS IS THE most common crippler in the United States. It affects one in every seven people. Only heart disease puts more people on work disability. In fact, back and joint problems account for over half of all visits to the family doctor, and they cost our economy more than $86 billion and 45 million days lost from work every year. If you don't get treatment, some forms of arthritis can leave you deformed, incapacitated, and even cost you your life.

A quick search through one of the major medical news sites on the Web will turn up over 47,000 articles on arthritis published in scientific journals over the past ten years, and if you Google the search terms "arthritis, alternative medicine," you'll get nearly nineteen million results.

That's a lot of information—too much for most of us to handle, *especially when so much of it is questionable or misleading*. Yes, that's right. Much of what people believe about arthritis just isn't true. Here are some common ideas about the condition, every one of them a myth:

Myth #1: Arthritis is a disease of aging. Anyone at any age can get arthritis. Half of my patients at the Arthritis Institute of Long Island are under age forty-five.

Myth #2: A cold, wet climate causes arthritis. Arthritis comes in many shapes and guises, but none of them are caused by cold, wet weather. Neither is a hot, dry climate a cure, although it can sometimes help. People feel better in warm, stable conditions not because of the temperature but because of the atmosphere's slightly higher and steadier barometric pressure. That's also what tells people with arthritis when it's about to rain. Before a storm, the barometric pressure falls, joint tissue swells, nerves stretch, and pain flairs up.

Myth #3: Arthritis can be cured. This myth has sent many people running for folk remedies that often prove useless and sometimes downright dangerous. There is currently no known cure for arthritis. However, there are ways of controlling its causes and symptoms, and in the case of rheumatoid arthritis, even of reversing the disease, if it's caught early enough.

Myth #4: Arthritis just means a few minor aches and pains. This myth has perhaps caused more damage than any other because it trivializes and dismisses the condition as a nuisance. The fact is that arthritis can be—and often is—devastating, debilitating, and even deadly. Untreated rheumatoid arthritis has the same mortality as untreated advanced heart disease.

With so much contradictory and false information about arthritis confusing our perceptions of the disease, what *is* true about it?

Fire and Smoke

There are more than 150 forms of arthritis, and each has its own, unique profile. On the surface, some seem no more similar than circles and squares. Why, then, do we classify them together? Because they all have one thing in common, a hallmark symptom that can lead to pain and disfigurement: *Joint Inflammation.*

That may not square with what you've heard. Many, if not most, people believe that the word arthritis is simply another way of saying "tissue breakdown in the joints." While that's true as far as it goes, it portrays only the end-stage of the disease—like describing a house fire as a pile of charred wood and smoking ashes. It misses the point. Broken down cartilage is like charcoal. Inflammation, on the other hand, is the body's version of roaring flames, and it can be nearly as destructive. Recent research has implicated inflammation in many diseases, including heart and circulatory ailments, cancer, asthma, allergies, autoimmune conditions, and of course, arthritis.

So exactly what are we talking about when we talk about inflammation? Fundamentally, it's just like that ordinary irritation you see (and feel) with an infected toe or a burn—and it's not always a bad thing. In fact, it's one of the first responses of your immune system to an attack by *pathogens*—destructive organisms such as bacteria or viruses that invade your body—or to anything else that damages body tissues, and it actually helps protect you. Here's how.

An inflammatory response consists of four components:

- redness
- heat
- swelling
- pain

Redness and heat occur because blood vessels downstream of an infection or irritation begin to narrow, causing blood to back up, fill, and expand the vessels upstream, as if you were crimping a hose. All that pressure then forces blood plasma (the liquid part of blood) to seep out of tiny, secondary vessels (capillaries) into surrounding tissue, making it swell. The swollen tissue, in turn, stretches nerves and pushes against them, causing pain.

When plasma leaks out of capillaries into surrounding tissue, white blood cells (*leukocytes*) and other types of immune cells go with it. They're then free to do their job of attacking and ingesting foreign organisms, cleaning up dead-cell debris, and walling off infection so that it doesn't spread. This type of inflammation is usually a good thing.

Problems occur when inflammation lasts too long. The first immune cells to rush to the site of an infection or irritation can survive for only a

MAKING LIFE A LITTLE EASIER

Long flexible shoehorns make getting dressed much easier. They usually start at seventeen inches and go up. These inexpensive aids are indispensable for putting on shoes if you have problems bending.

couple of days. If the problem hasn't been resolved by then, stronger, longer-lived cells called *macrophages,* take their place. If the irritation becomes chronic, these tough guys can hang around for weeks, months, or even years, using powerful poisons to destroy threats to the body. Unfortunately, these poisons also destroy healthy tissue, resulting in further inflammation and sometimes even causing organs to stop functioning properly. If the tissue is located in or around your bone joints, for example, they can lose their ability to move freely back and forth or side to side.

It Ain't Necessarily So

Joint pain, of course, is often an early sign of arthritis. What complicates the picture is that it can also be a symptom of many other ailments and can fool people into believing they have arthritis when they don't. Even primary care medical doctors and orthopedic surgeons commonly make this mistake in diagnosis when they focus narrowly on the individual areas where symptoms appear rather than on the whole patient.

It's important to rule out alternative possibilities, such as a herniated disk, sciatica, nerve damage in the hands and feet from diabetes (*neuropathy*), fibromyalgia, infections, and a host of other conditions. Some, including thyroid disease and kidney disease, can be quite serious. And one liver disease in particular, hepatitis C, is becoming almost commonplace. How often this ailment is mistaken for rheumatoid arthritis almost strains belief.

Obviously, making a correct diagnosis is extremely important. In some cases, like recognizing the difference between a mushroom and a toadstool, it can mean the difference between life and death. So if you have joint pain, it's important to see a specialist who is trained to think in terms of your entire system, not just your joints. Most often, that would be a *rheumatologist.*

If you're having pain in the knee or hip, he or she will almost certainly begin your treatment with a complete exam, including x-rays and laboratory tests, to rule out other illnesses. If you do turn out to have another illness, you'll either be sent back to your primary doctor or directly to a different specialist. If you have very advanced arthritis with severe tissue breakdown in a joint, your rheumatologist may send you to an orthopedist, a surgeon who specializes in operating on and reconstructing joints.

On the other hand, if the disease hasn't progressed to the extreme—and in most cases it hasn't—he or she can treat it with a variety of options, including exercise, diet, supplements, and medications. Rheumatologists are trained to look at the whole patient and view joint pain as a symptom of a systemic problem, not just an isolated issue. His or her job is to try to keep you away from surgery and able to lead a normal and active life.

Osteoarthritis

The most common type of joint inflammation is *osteoarthritis (OA)*, which currently affects about twenty-one million Americans. More than any other form of the disease, physicians have thought of OA in terms of tissue breakdown, that is, like charcoal and ashes. The traditional theory states that this breakdown happens mostly because of mechanical wear and tear, especially as you get older and the joints produce less fluid to ease the friction of bone rubbing against cartilage—the cushioning tissue between them.

The broken-down tissue then causes inflammation and sometimes the formation of calcium lumps called bone spurs. Recent research, however, is convincing more and more doctors that OA starts as a chronic, low-grade inflammation, which leads to tissue breakdown, rather than the other way around. By the time it has destroyed cartilage, it has become an end-stage disease.

I've seen evidence of this myself. Over the years, many patients have come to me complaining of persistent knee pain. Often, they have already consulted an orthopedist and undergone MRIs and x-rays—all of which turned up no signs of destroyed cartilage. Almost inevitably, they have been prescribed physical therapy, which failed to work. Fortunately, I had a trick up my sleeve that these orthopedists didn't have: needle arthroscopy.

The needle arthroscope, an instrument about as wide as a small paper clip, uses fiber optics to give a firsthand view of the inside of a knee joint. At the Arthritis Institute of Long Island, we were among the first medical professionals on the East Coast to have the needle arthroscope, and it opened up a whole new world to us.

With it, I saw things that I and others had never seen before. Many of these patients with knee pain had normal MRIs and x-rays. To my surprise, most, if not all of them, had significant osteoarthritis!

During the procedure, I would wash out small bits of tissue from their knees and send them for laboratory analysis. The samples often turned out to be full of inflammation—a discovery that led me to understand in a very immediate way that early osteoarthritis was an inflammatory disease, not one of "the joint just wearing out."

We didn't know, of course, what was causing the inflammation, and frankly, we still don't. It could be due to mechanical problems in the joints, or it may happen as a result of some genetic predisposition or an environmental trigger such as a germ or a toxin. Perhaps the answer to this riddle will eventually lead us to a true "cure" for arthritis. Until then, however, treating the inflammation, in my opinion, is our best bet.

The Three Faces of Osteoarthritis

If you have OA, it's likely to concentrate in one of three areas of the body:

The end joints of your hands and feet, and your finger, thumb, and toe joints.   This form of the disease, also called *nodal* OA, is thought to pass from generation to generation through genes from the mother's side of the family. It typically appears as swollen tissue, and can eventually cause pain and deformity.

The hips, knees, and shoulders.   This type of arthritis, which often develops at the site of an injury or joint instability, is more degenerative than nodal disease. The first symptom is often pain, especially after use. You're likely to wake up in the morning feeling fine, and then develop gnawing aches as you exercise or move about.

The spine.   This type of OA, also called *spondylosis,* can cause degeneration of the cushion-like discs that act as shock absorbers between your spinal vertebrae, and bring about the formation of bone spurs on your vertebrae and the joints between them. The result can be chronic, debilitating back pain.

As any type of OA reaches an advanced stage, some of the cartilage in the affected joint can disappear completely, allowing bone to rub on bone. When the damage is this severe, the joint will try to rebuild itself, but its misguided efforts at repair actually cause bone scarring (*sclerosis*), making the joint even worse. Because you can't really rebuild cartilage, the best plan of attack is to prevent the destruction from happening in the first

UNTREATED OSTEOARTHRITIS

If osteoarthritis (OA) goes untreated, you'll not only suffer constant pain, but you may overcompensate and cause yourself even more consequences. For example, if you have arthritic inflammation in your right hip, you may have trouble rolling over when you lie down, and when you walk, you may start to favor the opposite leg so that you end up putting pressure on other joints, causing your back, as well as your left ankle and knee to hurt.

place by treating the inflammation early in the course of the disease—putting out the fire before it gets out of control.

Rheumatoid Arthritis

Rheumatoid arthritis (RA) is the second most common form of the ailment, and left untreated, it can ravage and horribly disfigure the body. It is not a disease of aging. In fact, it often flares up in younger patients, usually women between the ages of twenty and forty. The first signs can include flu-like symptoms, such as fatigue, fevers, and rashes, but it soon invades the joints—mostly those of the fingers, hands, wrists, toes, feet, and ankles, as well as the elbows and knees.

As with OA, there are three types of RA. With the first type, patients can get better in about a year. The second type is slow and indolent in its progression and can keep going for ten or twenty years. Then there's a third type, which is exceptionally aggressive. Everything just swells up, and the disease becomes markedly destructive.

Also like OA, rheumatoid disease is an inflammatory process, but it doesn't develop in quite the same low-key way. It usually starts when something triggers your immune system into marshalling its forces to mount a defense, but instead of setting their sights squarely on destructive outside invaders, your defenses begin hunting down healthy cells as well—an *autoimmune* reaction.

When it goes for the joints, RA specifically attacks the *synovium*, the protective membrane that lines and feeds the joint surfaces. Unfortunately, the inflammation that results causes a peculiar response: the synovium begins to grow and act like a localized cancer, penetrating into the joints and eating away at cartilage and bone. At first, it can cause morning stiffness, which will feel better after exercising or moving around—exactly the opposite of OA. But eventually, the joints become hot, red, and swollen, and the swelling itself can cause even more problems. If it presses on nerves in the wrist, for example, it can cause Carpal Tunnel syndrome. If it puts pressure on neck nerves, it can cause neurological problems and even result in paralysis.

And the news keeps getting worse. RA doesn't stop at the joints—it attacks the entire body system. It can damage your kidneys, skin, bone marrow, and eyes, and 40 percent of patients have inflammation around their lungs (*pleuritis*) or heart (*pericarditis*). Scarring in the lung as a result of inflammation can be deadly, and RA can accelerate coronary artery disease—which is also thought to be an inflammatory condition—leading to a heart attack.

The Causes of RA

As with OA, we don't really know what starts the fire where RA is concerned, but we do have some ideas. The most likely culprit is a particular type of virus called a retrovirus. HIV, the virus that causes AIDS, is one member of this family, although it's probably not the one implicated in RA. In any case, we think that that a retrovirus inserts some of its own genetic material into the cells of the synovium and starts releasing chemicals to its surface. That tricks the immune system into thinking that the synovium is a foreign object, and it starts making antibodies to destroy it. But by the time we get in to look for the cause, the virus itself already is gone and the only thing left is a little piece of its gene that's almost impossible to find.

There is another theory that the guilty virus has certain characteristics on its surface that are similar to those on the surfaces of normal, healthy cells, so when you're exposed to it, you start making antibodies that attack both the virus and your own tissue at the same time.

Again, we don't know which microbe is responsible, although both the measles virus and the Epstein Barr virus, which causes mononucleosis, are good candidates.

THE MANY FACES OF ARTHRITIS: FIFTH DISEASE

Not everything that looks like rheumatoid arthritis (RA) really is, and it's important to make the distinction, as treatment depends on accurate diagnosis. Fifth Disease, also called *erythema infectiosum,* is a case in point. Fifth Disease is a mild, contagious viral illness that usually appears in children between the ages of five and fifteen. It is called Fifth Disease because it is usually the fifth disease of childhood, occurring after mumps, measles, chicken pox, and rubella. Early symptoms can include a low-grade fever, exhaustion, and a bright red rash on the cheeks—all of which suggest RA or lupus—another form of arthritis. As the infection progresses, the rest of the body may develop a lacy rash that gradually fades. With kids, that's usually the end of the story. But adults can get the illness too, and those who do very often go on to develop swollen aching joints in their fingers, wrists, and knees. The aching usually occurs in the same joints on both sides of the body, so it's *symmetrical,* and lasts anywhere from days to months. Fortunately, over half of all adults have already had the disease in childhood, and it seems to be a one-time event.

The Emotions of Arthritis

Obviously, the sooner treatment for RA begins the better. To quote an old saw, "An ounce of prevention is worth a pound of cure." If we get to the disease early enough, we can slow it down or stop it, and sometimes even reverse the damage it's done. If we don't, on the other hand, the results can be extremely challenging, both physically and psychologically.

I recently had the difficult duty of trying to help a woman whose RA had percolated for years before she finally came to the Arthritis Institute of Long Island for proper treatment. We'll call her Sally.

The first time I saw Sally, she was 81 years old and made her home in an assisted living environment. Two things about her struck me immediately—she was wheelchair bound and her visible joints were terribly deformed. Large, firm lumps, called *rheumatoid nodules*, had formed on the tips of her elbows, and her fingers were all bent askew, as if each had been broken in the middle and pointed in some haphazard direction.

At first, I was tempted to scold her for allowing her disease to go for so long without treatment, but a few moments of chatting with her made me realize that she *had* been getting treatment—the wrong treatment. Until recently, she had been living in rural Vermont, where her family doctor treated her symptoms with pain medication but had done nothing to deal with the underlying disease.

She couldn't quite bring to mind the name of the medication she had been taking, only that she had been coping with her condition for as long as she could remember. By now, it could have been decades. There was nothing to do but try and determine exactly how much damage had been done to her joints. After her examination, I ordered x-rays.

The pictures didn't look great, but they were better than I expected. Her elbows, shoulders, and finger joints were almost burnt out—bone rubbing on bone—but not totally destroyed. We could probably take care of these joints with medication alone, but her hips and knees would need surgery. The problem was that they still showed signs of active disease— they were full of inflammation, and any attempt to repair them while they were in that condition would fail. She would have to undergo a course of anti-inflammatory medications before we could do any reconstruction.

I put together a treatment plan for Sally and at her next visit presented it to her. It included medication, dietary changes, surgery, and even some limited exercise. I assumed she would be happy to hear that we could get her back on her feet, improve her comfort level, and restore some of her ability to perform the activities of everyday life. I was wrong. She wasn't happy. In fact, she was reluctant to participate. And I shouldn't have been surprised because arthritis affects more than the body. It affects the psyche—the mind and the spirit—as well.

Any disease that either inflicts chronic pain or limits physical activity puts you at risk for depression. Arthritis does both of those things.

That's one reason (among many) that rheumatologists recommend lots of exercise for their patients. Study after study has established that exercise is an effective adjunct treatment to medication for mild to moderate depression. Studies have also shown that up to 20 percent of patients with rheumatoid arthritis suffer from a clinical depression requiring medication. It has been my experience that unless the depression is addressed, no amount of medication will be effective. In many cases, depression is only the beginning of the complex emotions that arthritis sufferers go through.

Sally's case was typical. She was in constant pain, she couldn't grasp or walk, and yet she refused treatment. Why?

For all of the discomfort her disease was putting her through, it was also giving her a subtle collateral benefit. She was getting lots of attention. She was constantly surrounded by family, nurses, and other caregivers, and they were all there for a single purpose: to meet her needs. With so many people willing to look after her, she felt little motivation to battle through a round of operations that were designed to improve her ability to look after herself. In the same way that kidnap victims can gradually become emotionally dependent on their abductors, Sally had developed a dependent relationship with her disease. After suffering for so long a time, she could no longer remember the joy and pride of being self-reliant.

There was nothing to do but ask her to keep an open mind and try the medications for a couple of weeks. If they made her feel better, maybe we could then revisit thinking about surgical options as well. If they didn't, she could always choose to stop taking them. She reluctantly agreed.

I also had the opportunity to speak with two of Sally's daughters who frequently visited and helped with her care. They were enthusiastic about their mother's treatment plan, not only because it would ultimately help her to feel better, but because it would relieve them of some of the burden of looking after her as well.

In the end, with their help, encouragement, and moral support, Sally decided to cooperate and follow her treatment plan. I was able to improve her illness to such an extent that she has agreed to undergo evaluation for further treatment, which we hope will free her from her wheelchair. Her case underscores the need to get the right kind of help as soon as you can. Although I was able to stop the course of her disease and treat her pain more effectively, there was no way to undo the damage to her hands and elbows, and surgery is no fun at any age.

Of course, the very best case scenario would be to prevent OA and RA from ever developing in the first place, but to do that, we would have to know who is most likely to develop these diseases. Is such a thing possible? In fact, it is.

CHAPTER

Who Is Vulnerable?

WHO IS MOST likely to develop arthritis, and more importantly, do you fit the picture? Or if you already have arthritis, is there any way to know if you're likely to see improvement once you go into treatment? The answer is yes . . . and no.

Talking about risk is a risky business. There are people in the world who have high cholesterol, high blood pressure, diabetes, a bad smoking habit, and the activity level of a houseplant, yet they live to enjoy a happy, ripe old age. There are others who seem to have everything going for them—healthful diet, no cigarettes, regular exercise, and great genes—yet they're struck down by a heart attack or stroke in their forties. Assessing risk is rarely an exact science with regard to any disease, including arthritis.

Then Why Bother?

Unless we can identify *biomarkers*—genes with telltale characteristics that predict the onset of arthritis (and we're close to doing just that)—we can't say for certain whether or not you'll develop OA or RA. But we *can* give you a pretty good idea. We can tell you, for example, that if you're over sixty-five, overweight, and smoke, you're much more likely to get OA of the knee than is a person of the same age who watches his or her calories and avoids tobacco. In other words, a much higher percentage of people who have those risk factors will get arthritis than will people who don't. It's like saying the kids in any kindergarten class are likely to catch colds during the school year. That doesn't mean that every child in every class will get sick, but there's an excellent chance that many, if not most, will end up with a runny nose, sniffles, and a cough.

So if we can't be exact in our predictions, why should you care about your risk factors for arthritis? Two reasons. The first is to put you on alert. If you know your risk is high, maybe you will pay closer attention to any symptoms that might appear and get to a doctor more quickly. The second is that *you may be able to lower your risk*. You can't do much about factors such as age or gender, of course, but you *can* reduce your weight or quit smoking. At least some of your fate is in your hands.

Below are some of the most common risk factors for the most common forms of arthritis.

Age

The simple process of getting older makes you more likely to develop many medical conditions, including heart disease, cancer, stroke, and—you guessed it—arthritis. That's not true of all varieties of the disease, of course, but it is for OA.

Only six out of a hundred people at age thirty have any arthritis of the knee, and merely half as many have arthritis of the hip. Past the age of sixty-five, however, nearly everyone shows some degree of joint damage on x-rays—a fact that should come as no surprise. By that time, the joints have undergone a huge load of mechanical wear and tear, which can lead to chronic inflammation. You already know what happens next. Being older, however, is not the only risk factor related to age. Being younger also has its perils.

Children, for example, can develop what is appropriately called *Juvenile Arthritis (JA)* at any time from birth through late adolescence. Like its adult counterpart, JA appears in many guises. There's a juvenile rheumatoid arthritis, a juvenile psoriatic arthritis, and a juvenile lupus.

THE MANY FACES OF ARTHRITIS: LUPUS

In many ways, lupus (systemic lupus erythematosus) resembles RA. It is an autoimmune inflammatory disease in which your immune cells may attack the connective tissue in many areas of your body, including your joints. Its symptoms include joint pain and swelling, skin rashes, kidney inflammation, and inflammation of the fibrous tissue that surrounds the heart. If you're in treatment, you may have to take anti-inflammatory medications, avoid sunlight to reduce the rashes, exercise to fend off muscle weakness, and take immunizations to protect against infections. Depending on your symptoms, your doctor may also prescribe anti-malarial drugs, which will help alleviate skin problems; drugs that suppress your immune system to further control inflammation; or blood thinners to keep your blood from clotting inside blood vessels. Although many people have the impression that lupus is generally fatal, the outlook for patients today is more optimistic than it has ever been. Although the disease can become quite serious in some people, the vast majority who develop the disease will go on to live a normal, healthy lifespan.

The presenting symptoms, however, may be somewhat different from adult varieties. They're more likely to begin with rashes, high fevers, or eye inflammations. And arthritis doesn't seem to slow kids down in the same way it does grown-ups. A child whose knee is extremely swollen and filled with fluid can often run, jump, and play as if nothing were wrong.

RA tends to attack young adults. It's not unusual for a woman to start noticing symptoms at around age thirty, although they can appear as early as eighteen. Arthritis of the spine, *ankylosing spondylitis,* almost always appears in men between the ages of seventeen and thirty-five. Lupus, another systemic inflammatory rheumatic disease, occurs most commonly in women between the ages of eighteen and forty-five.

The point? While age is a factor in arthritis risk, each type of arthritis is associated with its own age group. So no matter how young or old you are, if you feel stiff, sore, or swollen in the joints, take your symptoms seriously and see a rheumatologist. I cannot stress enough how important it is to get an early diagnosis.

Family History

As research shows, your genes play a major role in determining whether you will develop arthritis, and that applies to both OA and RA.

A 1998 British study of 616 pairs of female twins showed that genes are probably responsible for at least half of all cases of OA of the hip. A more recent study, also British, looked at more than 700 brothers and sisters of patients with severe knee arthritis. Even allowing for other risk factors, the siblings were more than twice as likely to have the disease as were people not related to an OA patient. In my own practice, I often see cases of hand arthritis that seem to come down from grandmother, to mother, to daughter.

Interestingly, not only can your genes make you more prone to developing particular types of OA, but they can also have a profound influence on how severe the disease will be. Doctors in Sweden have shown that identical twins are five times more likely than fraternal twins to have severe knee or hip OA. Since identical twins share identical genes, and fraternal twins do not, the genetic factor would seem to be very strong.

Although scientists don't yet completely understand the genetics of OA, they do have evidence that mutations—permanent changes in the way a gene is built—may be responsible for at least a quarter of all cases of OA.

Likewise, if you have a familial history of RA, you're more likely to develop it yourself. Researchers have identified at least one gene (HLA-DR4) that affects the immune system and seems to be associated with RA. However, not everyone who carries this gene develops RA, so it's likely that other factors are involved as well.

Finally, once you've had one autoimmune disease, the odds increase that you'll develop others, including RA. It's not unusual to find Hashimoto's thyroiditis, a very common condition that causes the immune system to attack and destroy the thyroid gland, in a patient who is also dealing with RA or lupus. I also see family clusterings of various autoimmune conditions. For example, I had one patient, Mary P., who had lupus, while her sister had a harmless autoimmune condition called Raynaud's syndrome, and her mother had multiple sclerosis. Most likely, they all carried similar genes that made their immune systems behave in unpredictable ways.

Gender

In general, the impact of gender on arthritis risk depends on the type of arthritis you're talking about. In OA, the risk is relatively evenly distributed between males and females. RA, however, occurs much more often in women (80 percent) than in men. To add insult to injury, women don't respond as well to treatment. According to one group of doctors who presented evidence at the Annual European Congress of Rheumatology, females undergoing therapy are less likely to go into remission, or even to see their symptoms improve. No one knows why this should be. Although hormones would obviously come under suspicion, they aren't the only culprits. Some other internal factors—or even something external in the environment—probably play an important role.

One reason we know so little about the disease is that we haven't been able to reproduce it successfully in lab animals. These animals, often mice or rats, offer many advantages over working in clinical trials with humans. For one thing, their lives are much shorter, so we don't have to wait decades to observe the course of a disease. For another, we can manipulate the genes of lab animals to see which changes help them and which harm them. Because we haven't had appropriate mice to study RA, we have had none of these advantages in our research.

Now, all that has changed. Scientists at the Mayo Clinic have developed a strain of mice that shows an immune response similar to RA in humans and occurs more often in females. Working with these animals may soon bring us a much better understanding of the role of sex hormones, both in regulating risk factors for RA and in affecting the course of the disease.

Weight

We can't change our genes, gender, or age, but we can certainly reduce our body weight, and that makes hips, ankles, feet, and especially knees, less prone to arthritis. In fact, according to evidence presented at a recent American College of Rheumatology Annual Scientific Meeting, even modest weight loss can dramatically reduce pain and make performing the normal activities of everyday life much easier.

The knees have to bear a huge amount of load over a person's lifetime, and being overweight increases that load dramatically. A long-term weight loss program at the Johns Hopkins Arthritis Center in Baltimore has shown that women in their fifties and sixties who lost fifteen pounds over four months in a program of diet, exercise, and lifestyle changes experienced extraordinary reductions in pain. In fact, their quality of life was so improved that they compared themselves to healthy adults who did not have arthritis. And they found these changes so motivating that most kept their weight down throughout the following year.

I've seen similar results with my own patients. Dorothy L., a fifty-four-year-old, had gained forty pounds five years earlier. She had been going through deep depression and anxiety after a divorce. She came into my office complaining that she could barely walk because of the pain in her knees and ankles. I put her on a plan of supplements, exercise, and anti-inflammatory medication. What really worked best for her, however, was the Arthritis Super Diet (see Chapter 8), which not only added anti-inflammatory foods to her meals, but also helped her lose twenty-eight pounds over the next six months. At her lighter weight, she felt almost no knee ache, the bounce returned to her step, and she was able to stop her medication. As an added bonus, she looked ten years younger.

Another question has come up recently regarding arthritis and obesity—one we don't yet have an answer for. You may think of body fat as an inert substance that clings to your muscles like peanut butter, but it's actually a very active organ, producing many hormone-like chemicals that in

RA AND THE FAT CONNECTION

Although no one has yet demonstrated a link between body fat and RA, it may be just a matter of time. Scientists at Washington University School of Medicine in St. Louis have demonstrated that certain types of fat cells cause systemic inflammation that does lead to other conditions, including heart disease and diabetes. These cells are those that congregate in your belly and give you an "apple-shaped" body. However, not all of the fat in your abdomen is to blame. We know this because doing liposuction to remove large amounts of fat just under the skin has no effect on inflammation. Instead, the effect is caused by *visceral* fat, which lies deep in the gut and surrounds the organs there. This type of fat produces a chemical called *interleukin-6 (IL-6),* which is secreted into a large vein that drains blood from the area. IL-6, in turn, causes levels of an inflammatory substance called *C-reactive protein (CRP)* to rise in the body. Again, no one has yet done a study to establish whether visceral fat is a risk factor for RA, but high CRP is a biomarker for the disease, so the day may be soon coming.

large amounts can have toxic effects. So in addition to the damage it causes mechanically, it is entirely possible that fat may increase inflammation of the joints through the chemical effects of the by-products it manufactures.

As I said, we don't yet have an answer to this question, but you don't need to wait for one. The fat you carry is one risk factor you can begin to influence today. Make a decision. Eat sensibly and exercise regularly. If you can reach and maintain a healthful weight, you'll reduce your chances of developing severe OA in your lower body joints, and if you already have OA, you'll improve your quality of life immeasurably.

Athletics

Sports injuries of the past are often the arthritis sites of the future. Injury causes inflammation, and as you know, inflammation causes joint tissue to break down. But that's not the only problem. Young athletes seem to go out of their way to make the situation even worse.

Take, for example, a kid playing football in high school who injures his knee and gets a small tear in the cartilage. His coach tells him to go out and deal with the pain, so our young halfback ignores his body's warning signals, takes his position back on the playing field, and irritates the joint even more. After the game, his knee fills up with fluid, which puts pressure on the cartilage and prevents it from receiving nutrients. If he sees an orthopedist, the knee may be tapped to drain off the liquid. It may also get a shot of cortisone, which will temporarily quiet both the inflammation and the pain. End result? The kid continues playing on his bad knee, even when he goes to college. By that time, however, the joint has become so painful that he can't walk on it unless he tapes it up. Because of the original tear, there's instability in the joint. It wobbles. In fact, it's the wobbling that causes inflammation, because surfaces are rubbing against each other, even if only microscopically. Another ten to fifteen years go by, and voila! He has severe OA.

The same thing can happen after repetitive stress, even if there is no obvious injury. Someone who jogs ten miles a day every day for twenty years, for example, is going to run into problems from constantly pounding on cartilage that is naturally becoming less resilient with age. So if you don't modify the way you exercise—walking instead of running, for example—you may do serious damage to yourself and end up with crippling arthritis.

Occupation

It's commonplace knowledge: People who work in occupations that stress particular joints are more likely to develop OA in those joints. Bricklayers and carpet installers often end up with OA of the knees. Furniture movers find themselves moving into retirement barely able to stand up because of arthritis from back and hip inflammation. People who constantly type are more likely than others to develop OA of the hand or Carpal Tunnel syndrome.

What may be less well known, however, is that certain occupations are also associated with RA. For example, more men who work as conductors, freight and transport workers, farmers and farm workers, pulp and paper mill workers, textile mill workers, and bakers will eventually develop the disease. Women see higher rates if they work as printmakers or process engravers. The reason seems to be exposure to various kinds of organic dust such as fertilizers, or mineral dust such as asbestos. Presumably, the dust causes chemical changes in the human body that incite the immune system into a chaotic uproar and trick it into attacking normal, healthy cells.

The other occupational hazard that can cause RA, however, is more perplexing—vibration. Workers exposed to repeated episodes of strong vibration over the course of their career are more likely to develop the disease. No one is quite sure why.

Although occupation may seem at first to be a controllable risk factor, it's obviously difficult to change jobs mid-career. In fact, for some people, it's completely unrealistic. Most should consider it only if they have several other strong risk factors for OA or RA.

Infection

You know that infections can invade your skin, your organs, and even the nails on your fingers and toes, but did you know they can also wreak havoc on your joints? Two types of infection can lead to your developing arthritis. With the first, *local* infection, germs invade the joint itself. We call this septic arthritis. It can happen as a result of a direct wound, or your blood may carry bacteria in from somewhere else in the body. For example, they may come from a skin infection, called cellulitis, somewhere near the joint.

Another common source is the large bowel. As people grow older, they sometimes develop *diverticulitis,* a condition in which pouch-like pockets in the intestine wall become inflamed or infected. If one of these pockets ruptures, bacteria flood into the gut and often the bloodstream. A third common source is the teeth. Although it happens rarely, dental work can put bacteria into the bloodstream. This can result not only in arthritic symptoms, but can actually cause a very dangerous heart infection called *endocarditis*.

No matter the source, infection in a joint constitutes a medical emergency and calls for immediate attention. If the culprit is staphylococcus bacteria, it can chew up the entire joint within days.

The other type of infection that can lead to arthritic symptoms is *systemic*—one that affects the entire body. Joints are a secondary issue. Lyme disease is a good example. The Lyme bacteria can spread to the brain, the heart, the skin, as well as the joints. Hepatitis can also present with joint symptoms. Rheumatic fever is the granddaddy of them all. It's caused by a protein, carried by the streptococcus bacteria, that incites an autoimmune response. It's actually a very fleeting kind of arthritis that goes from one joint to the next. So a patient may come in with a large amount of fluid on her knee, but three hours later, the knee looks normal and a hand is swollen.

The good news about risk of arthritis from infection is that we can usually treat the condition successfully with antibiotics.

Smoking

The bad news about smoking cigarettes just never seems to stop coming. It raises your risk of heart disease, a host of cancers, chronic lung disease, prematurely-aged skin, and now, arthritis. In fact, according to researchers, if you're a woman and you smoke, you double your chances of developing RA, even if you have no genetic risk factor. Not a pretty picture.

But that doesn't let men off the hook. If anything, the outlook is even bleaker for male smokers. Scientists in Japan looked over the results of sixteen studies, and they came away with a dire conclusion: Men who smoke have double the arthritis risk factor of women who smoke!

RA AND CAFÉ

Think you're doing yourself a favor by switching from caffeinated coffee to decaf? Maybe not. Scientists at the University of Alabama at Birmingham have determined that older women who consume four or more cups of decaffeinated coffee every day doubled their risk of developing RA. On the other hand, those who drank three or more cups of regular tea reduced their risk by 60 percent. We don't know why decaf would have this effect, but we do know that tea, especially green tea, contains powerful antioxidants, which may be what keeps the RA at bay.

Heard enough? There's more. Doctors at the Mayo Clinic tell us that cigarettes not only increase your risk of RA, but they can worsen the damage done by OA as well. In looking at a group of male patients, they discovered that smokers had up to two-and-a-half times the risk for cartilage loss in knee OA when compared with the men who had previously quit smoking or had never smoked. Not only that, the smokers experienced much more pain.

How, you might wonder, could cigarette smoke possibly affect the knee joints? There are several possible explanations. Chemicals from the tobacco could make it difficult for new cells to form in the cartilage. They might also cause more free radicals to form and make mischief in the joint. Since smoke raises carbon monoxide levels in the bloodstream, it might also starve the cartilage of oxygen, thereby making repair difficult.

The Biggest Risk Factor of All

Being overweight is actually only one aspect of a larger risk factor, and it's one you can change: your diet. In fact, controlling what goes into your system may be the single most important thing you can do to relieve the symptoms of arthritis. The rules are simple . . .

Noshing and Gnashing

YOUR JOINTS, LIKE every other part of your body, depend upon good nutrition for good health. In fact, if you were to ask what magical ingredients should go into a perfect arthritis remedy, I would probably have to say, "Wild salmon with Dijon mustard, thyme, lemon juice, and turmeric." The mustard, thyme, and lemon juice are for taste. The turmeric and salmon, however, contain powerful anti-inflammatory nutrients that can put the pain of your arthritis on a very short leash. As an added bonus, this particular remedy can also help prevent heart attacks and strokes by keeping the lining of your arterial walls clear of dangerous inflammation and cholesterol deposits. And in reasonable doses, it has no known side effects.

You are—as they say—what you eat, so the more healthful your diet, the healthier your joints.

Good Guys and Not-So-Good Guys

What constitutes a healthful diet? For one, it's an eating regimen that keeps your body working the way it should. It makes your engine run smoothly without clogging your pipes or polluting your system. It doesn't pack on pounds of fat, but it does make you feel sated and satisfied. It helps you fight disease, heal, and grow new tissue. And it can help control inflammation.

MAKING LIFE A LITTLE EASIER

For chopping garlic, nuts, or seeds, use an electric spice grinder. These are inexpensive (between ten and twenty-five dollars) and can make chopping a quick, easy, and painless job.

Sounds like a tall order, but food can—and should—really do all that. If you tried to handle that many jobs with medications, you would have to swallow fistfuls of pills every day. That's because each medicine, no matter how powerful, has a specific, very narrowly defined task to perform. One pill, one result. Every food, on the other hand, contains a bouquet of nutrients, including proteins, fats, carbohydrates, fiber, vitamins, and minerals, that either singly or in combination can address many of the body's needs at once. Fruits and vegetables also contain *phytochemicals,* compounds that may offer extra disease-fighting effects.

Unfortunately, eating to control your arthritis isn't simply a matter of sitting at a banquet table and enjoying the feast. Not all foods are created equal. Some are anti-inflammatory, and some are not. A bag of potato chips, for example, isn't going to help you control your joint pain. In fact, it might actually make the pain worse because it contains *pro-inflammatory* substances—the guys we want to avoid. The first step in eating right, then, is learning how to tell the good guys from the not-so-good.

The Pro-Inflammatory Twins

We can divide foods that promote inflammation into two broad categories: unfavorable fats and unkind carbs. Here are some things to know about them:

Unfavorable fats are any fats that remain solid at room temperature. The list includes *saturated* fats, such as those you find in meats, dairy products, and some vegetable oils, such as palm and coconut. It also means *trans fats (trans fatty acids),* which are *unsaturated* fats with hydrogen added. Unsaturated fats, which usually come either from olives, peanuts, corns, cottonseeds, sunflowers, safflowers, or soybeans, are normally liquid at room temperature, but the hydrogen allows them to solidify. Major sources of trans fats include baked goods, margarine, shortening, some frying oils, and any processed food that contains the word "hydrogenated" among its ingredients. The problem with all of these fats is not so much that they're inherently "bad," but that they contain two types of inflammatory fatty acids, called *omega-6s* (particularly one called *arachidonic acid,* which plays a major role in arthritis) and *omega-9s*, that we generally eat far too much of. You can't eliminate these fatty acids from your diet altogether, and you shouldn't. You need small amounts for good health. But you need to balance them with another type of fatty acid, omega-3, which is anti-inflammatory. We'll talk more about omega-3s further on.

MAKING LIFE A LITTLE EASIER

When chopping garlic, let it sit for 15 minutes before using. This will allow the enzymes to reach full anti-inflammatory power.

By the way, here's a note of caution: Many people eat poultry and cold water fish such as salmon because they're supposed to be healthful. That's true for free range chicken and wild salmon, because they feed on foods that are low in omega-6s and high in omega-3s. Farmed chicken and fish, however, are a different story. They generally subsist on a diet that is high in omega-6s, and if you eat them, they'll pass those fatty acids on to you.

Unkind Carbs.   Carbohydrates are compounds that come from plants. Our bodies can turn them into a simple sugar called glucose, which our cells then use for energy. Unkind carbs are those that cause the volume of glucose in your blood to rise way too fast and way too high. All that glucose sends a signal to your pancreas to release a hormone called insulin into your bloodstream, which then tells your cells to soak up any nearby sugar. This brings your glucose level down to normal again. Here's the problem: When you have very high insulin levels much of the time, your cells start to ignore the signal to soak. They start to become *insulin resistant.* It's like the way most people react to noise. If you're sitting in a quiet room, the sound of a pin dropping can startle you. But if people crowd into the room and make a racket, you soon begin to tune it out.

The body's response to insulin resistance is to churn out more insulin. Eventually, the pancreas can work so hard at trying to get the cells' attention that it becomes exhausted and stops producing insulin. The result is Type II diabetes. That's why high insulin levels are associated with the development of diabetes, as well as obesity, and—you guessed it—inflammation.

The challenge, then, is to know an unkind carb when you see one. We used to identify them solely by their *glycemic index (GI),* which is a number that represents how fast and how high your blood sugar spikes after eating any particular food. But that number doesn't take into account the amount of carbohydrate in the food. The theory is that a small amount of unkind carbs (called *simple* carbohydrates in medical jargon) will have roughly the same effect on the body as a large amount of kinder carbs (called *complex* carbohydrates), which have a slower, milder effect on blood glucose. Nowadays, it's common to take a food's GI and multiply it by the amount of carbs it contains. The resulting number is called the *glycemic load* (GL). A GL between one and ten is considered low, between eleven and twenty moderate, and over twenty, high.

Does distinguishing between a food's GI and its GL really make a difference? It does. Watermelon is an often-cited example. Although the carbs in watermelon have a pretty high GI, most of the fruit consists of water, so the total amount of carbs in a slice is fairly low. If you looked only

A SPECIAL CASE: THE NIGHTSHADES

Although vegetables are generally very healthful, there are some that can present a problem for certain sensitive individuals: the nightshades. This group of plants includes foods—such as tomatoes, potatoes, eggplant, bell peppers, and hot peppers—and non-foods—such as tobacco, belladonna, and morning glory. All of them contain varying amounts of alkaloids, substances that can interfere with your nerve, muscle, digestive, and joint functions. In fact, some nightshade non-foods contain so much alkaloid that they're deadly poisonous, which is why you may have heard belladonna referred to as "deadly nightshade." Foods in this family, however, have relatively low alkaloid content, and cooking reduces the amount even further, so they're generally safe. Rare individuals, however, seem to have unusually strong reactions to these plants, so despite the obvious health benefits a tomato may have for most of us, nightshade sensitive people should avoid them.

at the GI, you might conclude that you should avoid watermelon at all costs, but the GL lets you know that it's actually a perfectly good addition to your diet.

Avoiding foods with a high GL is fairly simple. You don't really need a list to identify them (although if you want one, the most comprehensive GI/GL list ever compiled was published in the July 2002 issue of the *American Journal of Clinical Nutrition* and can be found online at www.ajcn.org/cgi/content/full/76/1/5. Just stay away from the following:

- Processed sugars
- Processed grains
- Processed cereals

Most 'white' foods, such as milled flour, pasta, and white rice, fall into one of these categories. Unfortunately, potatoes are also on the list, even if they're not processed. So is corn.

The Right Stuff

If it's important to keep your plate clear of unfavorable fats and unkind carbs, it's even more important to replace them with lots of favorable and kinder foods. The good news is that we can replace bad fats with good fats, bad carbs with good carbs, and maintain a diet that is not only healthful, but delicious as well. Here's what you need to know:

Favorable Fats, as mentioned above, contain omega–3 fatty acids. These acids produce a powerful anti-inflammatory action in the body. Not only can they help you control the pain and progression of your arthritis, but some scientific studies have suggested they may also help keep your heart healthy by suppressing inflammation and blood clotting in your blood vessels, reducing your cholesterol levels, lowering your blood pressure, slowing the growth of fat deposits on your artery walls, and preventing abnormal heart rhythms. As for their effects on arthritis, researchers have recently shown that they have benefits as strong as most non-steroidal anti-inflammatory drugs such as aspirin, ibuprofen (Advil, Motrin, Nuprin), naproxen sodium (Aleve), and others. That goes for both RA and OA.

Omega–3s come in three forms: eicosapentaenoic acid (EPA), docosahexaenoic acid (DHA), and alpha-linolenic acid (ALA). The body can only utilize the first two, EPA and DHA, to promote good health, but nature has given us a neat little trick: we can ingest ALA and turn it into EPA and DHA.

Although the news about omega–3s is generally positive, there are some risks if you take too much—more than three grams a day, according to the US Food and Drug Administration (FDA). We know, for example, that Inuit (Eskimo) people have very low rates of heart disease, probably because they eat lots of whale fat and seal fat, which contain high levels of omega–3. However, they also have an unusually high occurrence of hemorrhagic strokes—the kind that result from a blood vessel leaking blood into the brain. The FDA lists five main risks:

(1) increased bleeding times;

(2) the possibility of hemorrhagic stroke;

(3) oxidation of omega–3 fatty acids forming free radicals (that can damage cells);

(4) increased levels of low density lipoproteins (LDL) cholesterol (the kind that cause problems for your circulation); and

(5) reduced control of blood glucose levels among diabetics

Also, don't eat a lot of omega–3 foods if you have congestive heart failure, recurring chest pain, or any condition that may prevent your heart from getting enough blood flow.

One of the best sources of omega–3s is fish, especially fatty varieties that live in cold water. However, if you want to make fish a regular part of your diet, you may need to consider its mercury content. Unfortunately, mercury pollution remains a consideration in seafood generally, and more so in some species, such as tuna and mackerel, than others. While many adults can safely consume most fish three or four times a week, pregnant women, who can pass mercury on to a fetus, may have to be more careful. Experts generally consider salmon a safer choice than tuna or mackerel, although farmed salmon often contains relatively high levels of cancer-causing substances called PCBs—yet another reason to stick with the wild variety.

Here are some excellent sources of omega–3s:

- Cold water, oily fish (wild salmon, cod, tuna, trout, mackerel, herring, sardines, halibut)
- Flaxseed (ground into meal) and flaxseed oil
- Walnuts and walnut oil
- Canola oil (rapeseed oil)
- Pumpkin seeds and pumpkin seed oil
- Free range chicken
- Free range beef
- Broccoli

WHY SOY ISN'T ON THE LIST

Many "experts" would put soy right at the top of their list of anti-inflammatory foods, and in one respect, they would be right to do so. Soy does seem to reduce inflammation. However, there are health trade-offs involved, and I'm not sure they're worth making, given that so many other powerful anti-inflammatories offer the same benefits without posing similar risks. The problem is that soy contains substances called *isoflavones* and *phytoestrogens* that weakly mimic the action of the female hormone estrogen in the human body. Just as estrogen can fuel certain cancers such as malignant breast tumors, isoflavones (and in particular one called *genistein*) may do something very similar. The research has been contradictory. Some studies show soy may actually help prevent breast cancer, while others show the opposite may be true. We do know that in some Asian countries, where soy is a very common food, women are six times less likely to develop breast cancer. However, we don't know if that effect is because of soy or in spite of it. In any case, because the research is inconclusive concerning the safety of consuming high amounts of soy products, I don't include it on my list. Stick with cold water fish and flaxseed.

- Pinto beans
- Navy beans
- Kidney beans
- Chia
- Purslane
- Lingonberry
- Hemp

Kindly Carbs.   Despite what some diet gurus might tell you, carbohydrates are necessary for good health. In fact, they are the fuel your body runs on. As mentioned above, you want to avoid those that raise your blood sugar level too high and too quickly, but that still leaves a huge va-

riety of choices for your anti-inflammatory diet. There are two simple
rules to follow:

Rule 1: Choose whole grains.   And pass on the finely milled white
flour. Why? A whole grain consists of three parts. The first is an outer hull
called *bran*, which contains lots of fiber and is also a good source of vitamins B1, B2, and B3, as well as iron, zinc, magnesium, and phosphorous.
The second is the *germ*, rich in the same nutrients plus vitamin E. If you
planted the grain, which is actually a seed, a new plant would grow from
the germ. The rest of the grain is made up of the *kernel* (also called the *en-
dosperm*), which is where the carbohydrates are stored. The milling
process separates the three parts and discards the bran and germ, leaving
the carbohydrates in the starchy form you know as white flour. White
flour, as mentioned above, will make your blood sugar level rapidly
spike—exactly what you don't want. Whole wheat flour, on the other
hand, slows everything down because it still contains lots of fiber, which
protects the carbs from rapid digestion.

By the way, it's now easier than ever to choose whole-grain foods from
your supermarket shelf. In 2005, Oldways and the Whole Grains Council

FLAXSEED: A DOUBLE ADVANTAGE

Not only is flaxseed an excellent source of omega–3 fatty acids, but it also
contains a large amount of fiber as well. Just two tablespoons a day provides
139 percent of the amount recommended by the US Department of Agriculture.
One caveat, however: you need to use flax ground into meal. Whole seeds are
indigestible. Some people develop gastrointestinal symptoms, such as excessive
gas and bloating when they first add flaxseed to their diet. Although you can
safely add two tablespoons of ground flaxseed to your diet every day, it might be
wise to start with a smaller amount, say one teaspoon, and gradually add a little
more each day until you reach a full daily dose. Also, as with any soluble fiber, be
sure to drink plenty of fluids along with them.

created a stamp that clearly marks a product as containing either eight grams (50 percent) or sixteen grams (100 percent) of whole grains per serving. Currently, more than 800 products use the stamp on their packaging. Oldways is a nonprofit, food issues advocacy group. The Whole Grains Council includes chefs, scientists, and representatives from the food industry who work with Oldways to promote consumption of whole grains for better health.

Whenever you shop for whole grain foods such as breads and breakfast cereals, take some time to read the ingredients. If you see the words "sugar," "fructose," or "corn syrup" in the list, move on to another product.

SURPRISING POMEGRANATES

The pomegranate has been with us since the earliest days of human history. Farmers cultivated them in Egypt before the time of Moses, and it was known in India for at least as long. Recently, these sweet/tart fruits have found their way into medical research with surprising results. Scientists have discovered they may help prevent prostate cancer, heart disease, and diabetes. And according to a study done at Case Western Reserve University School of Medicine, they can also slow down the progression of OA. In the study, an extract of pomegranate was applied to tissue samples of human cartilage inflamed by osteoarthritis. The extract protected the cartilage against the ravages of interleukin–1b, a pro-inflammatory protein that plays a major destructive role in the course of OA. No one knows if simply eating the ruby red seeds of the fruit will be as effective, but it certainly wouldn't hurt to give it a try!

Rule 2: Choose brightly colored vegetables.   Look for brilliant reds, exuberant yellows, deep greens, and luscious oranges. The same is true for fruits. The more colorful they are, the more *phytonutrients* they're likely to contain. Phytonutrients, sometimes called phytochemicals, are substances found in edible plants that aren't exactly necessary for good health but can really contribute to it by fighting inflammation and disease. One way they do this is by acting as *antioxidants*. When oxygen combines with molecules in your body, the process produces *free radicals*, which are unstable chemicals that can cause untold mischief to your tissue. It's the same process that causes iron to rust and butter to turn rancid. Basically, free radicals go looking for other molecules to bond with. They're like bad dancers, pulling partners onto the ballroom floor, then stepping all over their feet. As you can imagine, inflammation is often the result. Antioxidants, such as those that come from phytonutrients, allow themselves to be chosen first, thus saving your tissue from some very bad treatment. Here are some great sources of phytonutrients:

- Blueberries
- Raspberries
- Strawberries
- Cranberries
- Pomegranates
- Apples
- Boysenberries
- Broccoli
- Kale
- Cauliflower
- Cabbage
- Brussels Sprouts
- Bok choy
- Winter squash
- Tomatoes
- Carrots
- Spinach
- Collards

- Onions
- Green tea

By the way, although the phytonutrients in food may help to keep arthritic inflammation under control, there's not much evidence that they have the same effect when delivered in supplement form. Anyway, pills and capsules make for terrible salad ingredients. Get your phytonutrients at the produce market, not the drug store.

One more tip: Eat fruits as soon as they ripen. If you let them sit longer, they'll produce more and more sugar, which will drive up their GL.

CHERRIES FOR ARTHRITIS?

The argument has been going back and forth since the first research was published in 1950 on the effectiveness of eating cherries as a remedy for arthritis. We would certainly all like it to be true, but is it? We do know from laboratory studies that substances found in cherries, called *anthocyanins*, can stop the body's production of certain enzymes that contribute to inflammation. We also know that tart cherries contain high amounts of melatonin, a powerful antioxidant. What we don't know is if simply eating cherries will actually relieve arthritis. The study in 1950 seemed at first to suggest that they can help alleviate not only the inflammation of arthritis, but of gout—another arthritic disease—as well. Scientists now agree that cherries can help alleviate the pain of gout, but they're still unsure about other forms of arthritis. The US Food and Drug Administration agrees: cherry growers will have to supply more proof before they can publicly claim that their favorite fruit is a powerful weapon in the fight against arthritis.

The Spices of Life

People often think that a healthful diet has to be bland. Nothing could be further from the truth. In fact, some spices take their place among the most powerful anti-inflammatory foods that we know of. Below are some examples. You can use any of them to liven up the taste of food, and many are available in pills or capsules as well. If you take them in supplement form, remember to follow dosage and instructions and cautions on the label.

Ginger.   Many studies over the past quarter-century have demonstrated ginger's anti-inflammatory properties, including one at the University of Miami that specifically concluded that *gingerols*, the active substances in ginger, work as well against OA of the knee as non-steroidal anti-inflammatory drugs like aspirin and ibuprofen. Even better, ginger doesn't have the same side effects as these drugs. Rather than upset your stomach as aspirin can, ginger can actually help settle it, and it's a great preventative for motion sickness. Ginger is also a wonderful addition to most shrimp, fish, and chicken dishes. By the way, commercial brands of ginger ale contain little or none of the spice, so they're obviously not a good source.

Turmeric.   Healers in India have used this member of the ginger family to reduce inflammation since ancient times, and modern scientific studies have confirmed its effectiveness. It's also a delicious ingredient in many curries and adds a yellow color to food. The active ingredients in turmeric are substances called curcuminoids, which act by switching off a pro-inflammatory protein (called NF-TK) in the joints. In one study at the University of Arizona, turmeric completely prevented the development of RA in lab animals. Because of the way it works, medical researchers hope it will also prove effective against other inflammatory disorders, including multiple sclerosis, asthma, and inflammatory bowel disease. It also shows some promise in the prevention of osteoporosis.

Cinnamon.   Some time ago, researchers demonstrated that cinnamon could help lower blood glucose, lipid, and cholesterol levels. Now, at least three new studies have shown that it can also help alleviate inflammation by controlling a protein that triggers the inflammatory response. Sprinkle it on your cereal, toast, or coffee now and then, but don't overdo. Cinnamon doesn't dissolve in water, so it has the potential to build up in the body. No one is yet certain what effects that might have. You may also want to take it in capsule form, so that it bypasses the saliva in the mouth on its way to the stomach. Saliva can actually reduce the beneficial effects of this spice.

Basil.   This is another herb that has been used for centuries in Asia to treat inflammation. Basil contains significant amounts of a fatty acid called *linolenic acid,* which powerfully reduces the effects of arachidonic acid, an omega–6 that is responsible for much of the pain and inflammation of OA. There is some concern about this herb, because it contains a compound called *estragole,* which may be a carcinogen and may cause uterine contractions. Estragole is present only in very small amounts, but still, I would caution against its use if you're pregnant or breast-feeding. Basil tastes great in tomato sauces, but you can also sprinkle it over fish and chicken dishes to add some zest.

Chives.   Like its cousins, onions, garlic, scallions, and leeks, chives are a member of the lily family and contain a powerful anti-inflammatory *flavonoid* (a plant pigment that is also a phytonutrient) called *quercetin.* Many laboratory studies, including a very recent one at Bordeaux University in France, have demonstrated that quercetin has a clear and strong effect in reducing the number of certain pro-inflammatory cells (*cytokines*) produced by the immune system. The result is less discomfort in the joints. Chives make an excellent ingredient in salads and can always be used as a garnish.

Folk medicine has also made use of other spices to reduce inflammation, although there is little scientific research either to support or disprove their effectiveness. These include:

- Cilantro
- Cloves
- Parsley
- Cardamom
- Black pepper
- Rosemary

Of course, in addition to spices, there are lots of over-the-counter remedies for arthritis sufferers. The big question is, which work and which don't?

Over the Counter

OVER-THE-COUNTER (OTC) supplements and medications can be good additions to your *Too Young to Feel Old* program. Some actually do help relieve pain and reduce inflammation. However, notice that I said, "good additions," and not "great additions." Too many people believe popping a few pills purchased at their local health food store or pharmacy will suddenly make all of their health problems vanish. Not true, and here is why.

Supplements Are Secondary

With the exception of multivitamins, most supplements are formulated around a single "active ingredient." That means that a capsule or pill contains only one biologically active substance, a vitamin or enzyme. These ingredients have either been extracted from some natural source such as a plant, or have been artificially manufactured. Here's the logic: If a tomato contains a powerful antioxidant such as a lycopene, why not just take doses of pure lycopene and bypass all the other unnecessary parts of the fruit? After all, you can concentrate a whole lot more of the enzyme into a capsule than you can into even a very large tomato.

Sounds like a good idea, but experience argues otherwise. Study after study has shown that consuming foods high in vitamin E such as nuts, vegetable oils, whole grains, tomato products, and dark-green leafy

MAKING LIFE A LITTLE EASIER

Put the kitchen items you use most often in easily accessible and reachable places. Keep frequently used utensils in upper drawers and dishes on the lower shelf of your cupboards. Coffee mug trees keep your cups close at hand for easy reach.

vegetables may lower your risk for cardiovascular disease and some cancers. Vitamin E supplements, on the other hand, have *not* consistently shown the same benefits, and some research suggests they can actually do harm. That may be because E-rich foods contain all three forms of the vitamin: alpha-tocopherol, gamma-tocopherol, and delta-tocopherol, whereas supplements usually contain only the alpha form. Or perhaps the benefits don't come from vitamin E alone, but rather from the combined effect of hundreds of complex chemicals found in each of these foods.

This last explanation actually makes sense from an evolutionary perspective. Throughout the history of our species, our bodies have learned to respond to whole foods, not isolated chemicals in those foods. We have complex relationships with what we eat. So the general rule is: Skip the beta carotene capsule, and drink fresh carrot juice instead.

General rules, of course, are made to be broken—at least occasionally. As I said before, some supplements and OTC medications *do* have a place in your daily anti-arthritis program, but only as an addition to the Arthritis Doctor's Super Diet (see chapter 8). Here are some I recommend—and a few I don't:

Calcium

Calcium intake is important. It is the most abundant mineral in your body, with nearly all of it stored in your bones and teeth. Not only does it help fight the ravages of arthritis, but it also helps prevent osteoporosis—a common side effect of both OA and RA. Unfortunately, dairy products are the richest dietary source of calcium, and that presents a problem, especially if you're trying to keep your caloric and fat intake down. If you were to depend on milk as your source, for example, you would have to drink two-and-a-half quarts a day. Even with skim milk, that's 850 calories a day. Who can do that?

ARTHRITIS AND OSTEOPOROSIS

Few people realize that osteoporosis is often a side effect of arthritis. This happens for many reasons, but primarily because of disuse of affected joints, along with poor nutrition and low calcium intake. An x-ray of an arthritic finger joint, for example, will often reveal thinning bone all around it because that finger is not being moved enough, and you need to have activity to keep bones strong and healthy. You also need plenty of calcium—a basic building block of bone. So remember to exercise and supplement!

Obviously, with this particular mineral, supplementation is a good idea.

You can buy calcium from your local health food store, pharmacy, or Internet site in two basic forms: Calcium citrate and calcium carbonate. Both have advantages and disadvantages. The carbonate form can cause constipation, but you don't have to take much of it because it contains lots of elemental calcium. The citrate form is usually easier to tolerate, but you have to take a bit more because it's not nearly so dense with calcium. Finally, it comes down to a matter of personal choice. You can get all the calcium you need from either form.

How much calcium do you need? I usually recommend between 1,500 and 2,000 mg of calcium every day. The FDA recommends 1,000 before age 50 and 1,200 after, but for post-menopausal women, it should be around 1,500. The Arthritis Doctor's Super Diet (see chapter 8) will give you close to 1,000 mg a day already, so you won't need to take much extra.

The least expensive calcium supplement I know of is the OTC heart-burn medication TUMS, which is composed totally of carbonate. Each tablet contains 500 mg. If you're on the Super Diet, take one TUMS a day. If you're on another diet that contains less calcium, take two tablets.

If you simply wish to add more calcium to your diet, eat more green leafy vegetables such as broccoli, collards, kale, mustard greens, turnip greens, and bok choy. Canned salmon and sardines can also be good choices, especially if they're canned with their bones. Significant amounts of calcium are also often added to commercially-made orange juice and bread.

Certain people shouldn't take extra calcium—those who have a history of kidney stones, those who have certain endocrine problems like hyper-parathyroidism, and those who have kidney disease.

Fish Oils

In the last chapter we discussed the importance of long-chain omega–3 fatty acids in fighting arthritis inflammation, and how cold water fish are the best source of these oils. Wild salmon is your best choice, but if the idea of salmon for dinner a couple of times a week doesn't appeal to you, then supplementing with fish oil is an acceptable second-best.

Fish oil generally comes in two forms: capsules and liquid. Soft gel capsules are okay, in that they don't need to be refrigerated and they're convenient, but at effective doses they tend to be pretty large and hard to swallow. More and more of my patients are taking the liquid fish oil by spoon instead of in capsules. Mind you, I'm not talking about the old-fashioned cod liver oil your grandmother used to force on everyone under the age of twelve. That stuff could gag a sword swallower and doesn't ac-tually contain the concentration of omega–3s you need. I'm talking about concentrated oil extracted from salmon, to which many manufacturers, such as Nordic Naturals and Carlson's, add a pleasant lemony flavor, mak-ing it very palatable.

I recommend at least 2000 mg a day of omega–3s to get a potent anti-inflammatory effect. That's two teaspoons of fish oil (or roughly 3 oz of fresh, wild Alaskan sockeye salmon). If you use soft gels, you need to check the label for dosage of omega–3 fatty acids per capsule. This can get a little tricky. Remember, you're not looking for the amount of fish oil in each capsule, but rather, the amount of essential fatty acids. The acids are called EPA (eicosapentaenoic acid) and DHA (docosahexaenoic acid). The total amount of both these acids combined will give you the number you're looking for. Also, be careful to distinguish the amount of omega–3s in a *serving* from the amount in a single capsule. Almost always, the amount of omega–3s listed on the label refers to one full serving, which often consists of *two* soft gels, not one. As you can see, getting your fish oil in capsules can be very confusing, and to make matters worse, they can be pretty expensive. So once again, your best bet is simply to take the oil by spoon.

Whatever brand you buy, you need to look for the words "mercury free" on the label. That's very important, especially for pregnant women.

Flaxseed Oil

Flaxseed oil is another good source of supplementary omega–3 fatty acids. In fact, it contains the highest omega–3 concentration of any vegetable. However, it contains only a *short chain* form, alpha-linolenic acid (ALA). In order to use short-chain omega–3s, the body must convert them into their long-chain cousins, EPA and DHA. Because of this, you'll need to take twice as much flaxseed oil as fish oil. That comes to two tablespoons a day. You should look for flaxseed oil that is cold-pressed and unrefined. I prefer filtered, but those who want more lignans and fiber should purchase the unfiltered brands. The two brands that my patients prefer are made by Spectrum Essentials or Barlean's Organic Oils, L.L.C. If you decide you'd rather supplement with flax meal, substitute a tablespoon for every teaspoon of fish oil.

MAKING LIFE A LITTLE EASIER

If you prefer to mill your own flaxseed meal from whole flaxseeds, shake the meal through a flour mill to remove the larger broken hulls.

Glucosamine and Chondroitin (C/G)

Volumes of praise have been written about the wonders of these two substances in treating arthritis. Unfortunately, very little of the praise is deserved.

Both compounds are found naturally in the body. Glucosamine is a form of amino sugar that may help form and repair cartilage. Chondroitin sulfate is part of a protein molecule that makes cartilage elastic.

What you purchase in supplement form comes from animal tissue. Glucosamine is extracted from shellfish shells; and chondroitin sulfate from cartilage—often shark cartilage or pig tracheas (so they're not Kosher or for the strict vegetarian).

Despite claims from manufacturers and enthusiasts that the C/G combination can slow and even reverse the joint damage done by arthritis, no credible study has come to the same conclusion. What research has in fact shown is that some people who take these supplements experience pain relief about equal to that experienced with non-steroidal anti-inflammatory drugs (NSAIDs) such as aspirin and ibuprofen.

If you want to use C/G supplements for simple pain relief, they may help, but even at that, they aren't very cost effective. Tylenol is far cheaper and works just as well. (I don't recommend NSAIDs because of possible side effects.)

Ginger Extract

Ginger root offers a wide variety of health benefits, among them motion sickness prevention, safe nausea relief for pregnant women, possible protection against ovarian and colorectal cancers, and of course, anti-inflammatory effects in the joints. We believe that these benefits come from compounds called *gingerols*, but again, rather than take a ginger extract that contains only these substances, you're better off adding ginger root to your cooking whenever you can. Not only are you more likely to experience all of the benefits ginger has to offer, but you'll also be more certain that you're getting what you're paying for. Because OTC supplement distributors don't come under the same scrutiny and control that pharmaceutical companies do, you can never be sure just how much—if any—of the ingredient on the label is actually in the product. Once again, a supplement may be an okay choice—better than no ginger at all—but it's certainly not the best.

Cinnamon

Cinnamon can be taken either in a capsule or added to food with equal effect. Why? Because cinnamon is never extracted. The capsules contain pure cinnamon powder, and that's helpful because eating a couple of teaspoons a day is difficult for most people, even if they add it to food. Cinnamon comes in two forms in the United States, Chinese and Ceylon. The Ceylon variety is a little sweeter and subtler in taste than its Chinese cousin, but both offer the same anti-inflammatory benefits. Cinnamon may also help control blood sugar in people with diabetes, prevent clots from forming in your bloodstream, and fight against infection, both bacterial and fungal.

MAKING LIFE A LITTLE EASIER

If you have trouble bending, make your cleaning easier when washing the bathtub. Sprinkle cleanser in the tub, and then use a clean long-handle mop to scrub. No bending!

Turmeric

Turmeric is a cooking spice—often used in curry—that has had a place in traditional Chinese and Indian healing since ancient times. Both its volatile oils and its bright yellow pigment, called curcumin, have powerful anti-inflammatory properties. In fact, laboratory studies have shown it to be as potent as hydrocortisone in relieving inflammation, but with none of the unpleasant side effects of the drug. In one particular study of patients with RA, curcumin shortened the time patients felt morning stiffness, allowed them to walk for longer periods, and showed marked reduction in joint swelling. Use 1.5 mg of turmeric root powder, either in food or a capsule, every day for best results.

Garlic

In my opinion, garlic is wonderful. Past studies have shown that it may have the ability to lower blood pressure and cholesterol levels; reduce atherosclerosis (plaques that stick to the inside walls of arteries) and arteriosclerosis (blood vessel stiffness); kill bacteria, viruses, fungi, and parasites; and even possibly protect against stomach and colon cancer. To be fair, there is controversy surrounding all of these claims. Some studies were poorly designed, and newer studies have sometimes given different results. The strongest evidence supports its lipid-lowering and anti-cancer effects. However, about one result there is little argument: garlic contains powerful antioxidants, which are important for your joint health.

Here is how it works: In the outer portion there's an enzyme called alliinase, which becomes active when the garlic is crushed. The alliinase converts alliin to allicin, an anti-inflammatory. After crushing, you have to let the garlic sit for ten or fifteen minutes. That allows it to develop more of the active ingredient. Using it right away doesn't allow it to reach its full potential. I'm not convinced about Garlique and odorless garlic capsules. Having it in its natural state is better.

The usual adult dosage is one to two cloves a day. In dried powder form, take 300 mg, two or three times a day, and aged extract, 7.2 grams a day.

Valerian Root and Melatonin

Both of these are popular sleep aids that mimic the action of natural hormones in the body, and patients with arthritis often have difficulty sleeping. Pain is one issue for them, and RA actually can actually trigger disturbances in the natural sleep cycle. So valerian and melatonin would seem like natural solutions to the problem. I have some concerns about both supplements.

Valerian does seem safe and effective for mild sleep disorders. There is evidence that it brings sleep on more quickly and helps the person reach a deeper state of slumber. But its safety has been shown only for short-term use—about two weeks—and at least one study suggests that people who use high doses of valerian on a regular basis over several months experience withdrawal symptoms similar to those caused by people withdrawing from any of a family of tranquilizers called *benzodiazepines (benzos)*. Symptoms for benzo withdrawal can include insomnia, anxiety, rapid heartbeat, high blood pressure, depression, tremors, excessive sweating, excessive dreaming, loss of appetite, and ringing in the ears.

Melatonin is a hormone produced by an organ in the brain called the pineal gland, so obviously the stuff in melatonin supplements doesn't come from human beings. It's artificially manufactured. This leads to the same old problem we see with many supplements: while we know that melatonin from your brain helps regulate sleep, there is very little evidence that supplements will do the same thing. And to be honest, I'm not entirely comfortable with anyone taking a hormone, artificial or natural, for a long time unless there is a long history of research into its safety and effectiveness. Melatonin can make allergies worse, interfere with post-puberty growth and development, neutralize the effectiveness of steroid drugs, and most importantly for our purposes, aggravate existing autoimmune disease. Since RA and several other types of arthritis are autoimmune in nature, I can't really recommend melatonin for supplementation.

SAM-e

I've known many people who take SAM-e thinking that it's going to cure their arthritis. It doesn't. Some lab studies suggested it might reduce inflammation, but I haven't seen it work with my patients. And no one seems yet to have unarguably demonstrated benefits from the supplement. In 2002, the U.S. Public Health Service published a summation of ninety clinical trials of SAM-e and reached no new definitive conclusions.

Vitamin E

Claims for vitamin E have ranged from improved virility to softer, suppler skin. In my experience, many people get headaches when they take it, and as I mentioned above, it doesn't seem very effective in supplement form. I also have some concern that, because it's a fat-soluble vitamin, it may have the potential to cause adverse liver problems.

Quercetin

Quercetin is a flavonoid that contains powerful antioxidants. It's what gives color to apple and onion skin, and it's also abundantly present in red wine, green tea, and St John's Wort. There is some evidence to show that quercetin can relieve the symptoms of allergies and asthma, prevent prostate cancer, and act as an anti-inflammatory, relieving pain in arthritic joints. Although as always I would rather see my patients getting their quercetin from food sources, its beneficial effects have been shown to occur with oral supplements. Doses range from 200 to 1,200 milligrams, and when taken by mouth, have shown no side effects. I recommend 500 mg a day.

> **MAKING LIFE A LITTLE EASIER**
>
> Wide rubber bands can be very helpful to people who have trouble gripping. Wrap them around doorknobs and drinking glasses to provide a better gripping surface.

White Willow Bark

This supplement certainly works. White willow bark was the first known source of salicylate, the active ingredient in aspirin. So why not just take aspirin? Quality control in the manufacture of aspirin is strict and precise, but with white willow bark, as with all supplements, what you pay for is not necessarily what you get—and it can be expensive. In any case, the same warning that applies to aspirin applies to white willow bark: People who have bleeding disorders, are on blood thinners, or have stomach ulcers shouldn't take it. It can cause profound bleeding problems.

Devil's Claw

Devil's claw is an extract from the root of a plant that grows in the Kalahari region in southern Africa. In Europe and the U.S., it's mostly used as an anti-inflammatory and pain reliever for joint problems. More and more studies are showing that devil's claw is safe and somewhat effective in treating osteoarthritis. Devil's claw does have some side effects: stomach upset, low blood pressure, and rapid pulse. You should also avoid using devil's claw if you have stomach ulcers or use blood thinners or aspirin. You can take 600 to 1,200 mg by mouth up to three times per day.

Cat's Claw

The cat's claw herb came originally from the Amazonian region of Peru, where it has been used to treat everything from cancer to infections. It's even used as a contraceptive. In the U.S., it's often marketed as an anti-viral remedy, but there hasn't been nearly enough research yet to substantiate those claims. Cat's claw comes in two varieties: *Uncaria tomentosa* and *Uncaria guianensi*. A small clinical trial had positive results for *tomentosa* in the treatment of RA, and another study showed *guianensi* to be effective in treating OA. Neither form showed any adverse effects. There is no established dosage for cat's claw, but it's widely available in many forms at health food stores and from the Internet, so I would recommend simply following the instructions on the label.

Primrose and Borage Oil

In the past, I have recommended primrose oil and borage oil, both of which are high in omega-3 fatty acids, but as it turns out, they're also high in omega-6 fatty acids, the bad guys, so I've taken them off my list of favored supplements. So should you.

Topicals

Topical anti-inflammatory creams or lotions come in two varieties: contra-irritants and trans-dermal transporters. Here are examples of both types.

Menthol.   Mentholated OTC topical pain relievers are contra-irritants, and they're great for temporary relief. They fool the nerve into thinking the skin is warm and that helps take away pain from the joint by fooling the brain into concentrating on the warmth. Menthol, by the way, is the only FDA-approved OTC contra-irritant.

Capsaicin.   This is another contra-irritant, which contains the active ingredient from hot peppers. Instead of creating warmth, it irritates the skin and confuses the pain nerves and thus takes pain away from the joint. The problem is that people just don't tolerate it well. It can cause nearly unbearable burning, and many times, since it's fat soluble—you've eaten hot pepper and you know how hot it is and how long it stays in your mouth— once it gets into the skin, it lasts a very long time. I don't recommend it.

Trolamine salicylate.   This is an odorless ingredient that has some pain-killing properties and actually penetrates the skin to deliver its effect. It is the only FDA-approved transdermal topical analgesic. This is the main ingredient in Aspercreme and similar products.

Emu oil.   This is a personal favorite of mine. It absorbs rapidly through the skin into fatty areas and it has omega-6 and omega-3 fatty acids in it. It's a great transport agent, so it's often used as an ingredient in products with pain relievers as well. My patients have had good success with it, and it's a personal favorite of my wife's as well because it makes her skin amazingly soft. Don't worry about dosage, just rub a little over the affected area.

CHAPTER

All-Important Exercise

Once upon a time, it was a commonplace idea in the medical community that exercise and arthritis were not a good match. Now we know better. The right physical activities can reduce joint pain and stiffness, strengthen muscles around the joints, increase flexibility and endurance, aid in maintaining full range of motion, and help you develop better balance. They can also improve circulation and help fight depression, and are indispensable to weight control.

The question, of course, is what sort of physical activity to do. Generally, exercises come in one of three distinct flavors: recreational and fitness, competitive, or therapeutic. We, of course, are interested in a therapeutic approach. The exercises will fall into four basic categories:

- Flexibility movements for range of motion. These include stretching exercises.
- Resistance movements for building strength. These are either *isotonic* (working against an outside weight such as a dumbbell) or *isometric* (working against your own strength, as when you push your hands against each other).
- Aerobic for cardiovascular fitness. These include walking, running, or any other movement that increases heart rate.
- Body positional for improving balance. These include posing or slow moving exercises like tai chi and yoga.

The exercises included in this chapter are mostly for flexibility/range of motion, although some will also help with increasing your strength and improving your balance. I don't particularly recommend that you do isometric exercises. Isotonic exercises, such as weight lifting or working against stretch bands, are okay, but in the beginning you should do them under the supervision of a therapist.

Getting Started

Twenty-nine exercises appear below, but you don't need to do all of them. Ten of them are core exercises (see box), which make up the Arthritis Doctor's Superset, the physical activity component of the twenty-eight day program. You should do these five or six days a week. You can add in any other exercises that are appropriate for the particular joints giving you trouble. If you can, perform the movements in front of a mirror to be certain you're doing them correctly. Also, wear comfortable shoes, and if you're using a piece of furniture for balance, make sure it's very sturdy.

A note of caution: Often, when people start an exercise program, they immediately go at it full force. Don't. It's probably the biggest mistake you can make. You'll end up sore and stiff the next day, and you'll most likely have to wait several days before you can pick up where you left off. My best advice is to start slowly, don't push yourself to the point of discomfort, and allow yourself at least a month to get up to speed. Here's a schedule to follow:

WEEK 1: Exercise no more than ten minutes a day, five or six days a week. Do one set of ten repetitions for each exercise.

WEEK 2: Increase your time to twenty minutes. Do two sets of ten repetitions for each exercise.

WEEK 3: Increase your time to thirty minutes. Do three sets of ten repetitions for each exercise.

WEEK 4: Add twenty to thirty minutes of brisk walking, three days a week, to your program. This will help improve your cardiovascular fitness.

If you have the time, you can also try yoga or tai chi, both of which have proven effective at not only improving overall fitness, but also at calming the mind and lifting the emotions. Tai chi, in particular, has undergone several studies that show it actually reduces falls among older adults, and as a side benefit, seems to strengthen the immune system as well.

Use particular caution if you've had any type of heart or lung disease or if you've had recent surgery. As with any exercise program, check with your own doctor before beginning this one.

THE ARTHRITIS DOCTOR'S SUPERSET

The following exercises should be done every day as part of your Arthritis Doctor's 28-Day Program:

Pip Finger Flexion (Page 74)

Wrist Flexion (Page 77)

Elbow Turns (Page 80)

Shoulder Abduction with Wand (Page 82)

Corner Stretch (Page 83)

Lower Back Stretch (Page 86)

Standing Hip And Knee Flexion (Page 95)

Standing Toe Raises (Page 97)

Neck Flexion and Extension (Page 99)

Neck Rotation Exercises (Page 100)

The
Exercises

Pip Finger Flexion

EXERCISE IS TO HELP WITH:
Grasping • Writing • Holding onto Eating Utensils

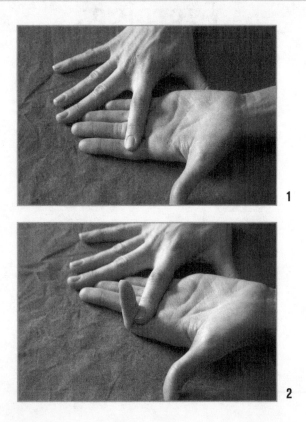

1

2

1. Place back of hand on a table with the palm side up (Figure 1).
2. Immobilize the lower knuckle (the MCP joint) with the forefinger of the opposite hand (Figure 1).
3. Bend the finger from the middle joint to 90 degrees (Figure 2).
4. Repeat exercise 10 times, for each finger of both the right and left hand.

Dip Finger Flexion

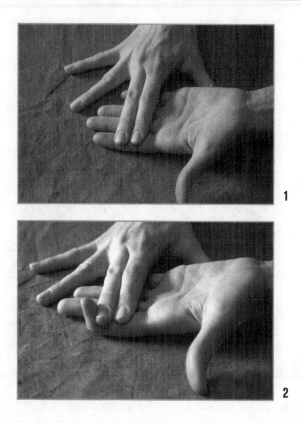

1

2

1. Place back of hand on a table with the palm side up (Figure 1).
2. Immobilize the middle knuckle (the PIP joint) with both the forefinger and the middle finger of the opposite hand (Figure 1).
3. Bend the finger from the end joint to 90 degrees (Figure 2).
4. Repeat exercise 10 times, for each finger of both the right and left hand.

Walk Your Fingers

EXERCISE IS TO HELP WITH:
Grasping • Playing Musical Instruments

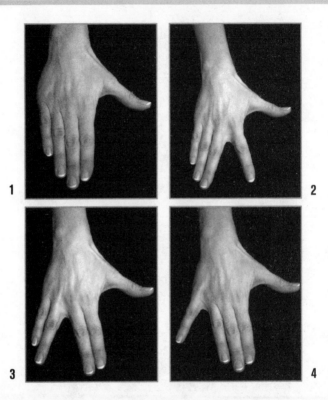

1. Rest your hand on a flat surface, palm down (Figure 1).
2. Move one finger at a time toward your thumb, starting with your index finger (Figure 2).
3. Lift and move your middle finger toward your thumb (Figure 3).
4. Lift and move your ring finger toward your thumb (Figure 4).
5. Finally, move your little finger toward the thumb.
6. Don't move your wrist or your thumb during this exercise. Repeat 3 times.
7. Repeat with the other hand.

Wrist Flexion

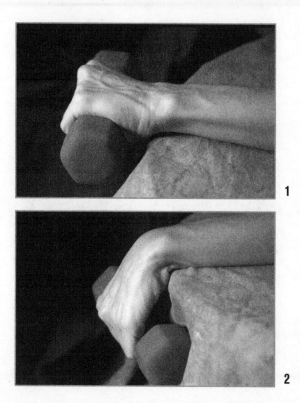

1. Rest the forearm comfortably on a table so the wrist lies just at the end of the table (Figure 1).
2. Hold a light weight in your hand; allow the wrist to slowly flex downward (Figure 2).
3. Count to 3 and slowly bring the wrist up so it is parallel to the table. Hold this position for a count of 3. It is important to keep your wrist just over the side of the table during this exercise.
4. Do both wrists, 10 times each.

Wrist Extension

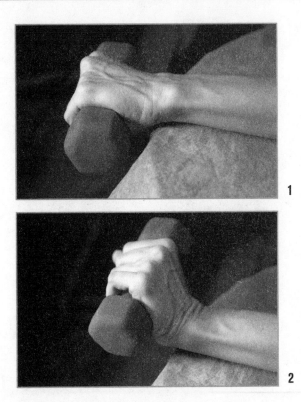

1

2

1. Rest the forearm comfortably on a table so the wrist lies just at the end of and parallel to the table. (Figure 1).
2. Hold a light weight in your hand, allow the wrist to slowly extend upward (Figure 2). Count to 3.
3. Slowly bring down your wrist so it is parallel to the table and in the starting position. Hold this position for a count of 3.
4. Do both wrists, 10 times each. It is important to keep your wrist just over the edge of the table during this exercise.

Radial and Ulnar Deviation

EXERCISE IS TO HELP WITH:
Reaching • Cutting Food • Using Tools • Fishing

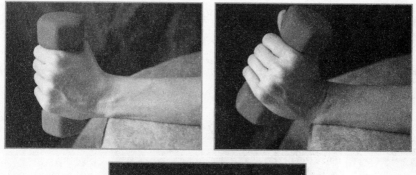

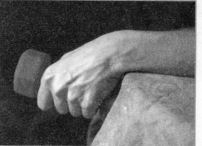

1. Sit with your forearm resting on a table with your wrist over the side. Have your hand in a "handshake" position (Figure 1).
2. Hold onto a light weight or a soup can.
3. Slowly bend your wrist up (Figure 2), hold it for 3 seconds, then bend your wrist forward (Figure 3) and hold this position for 3 seconds.
4. Repeat another 9 times.
5. Repeat the exercise with the opposite hand.

Elbow Turns

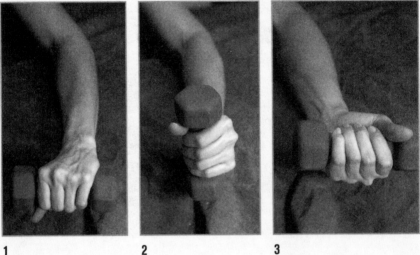

1   2   3

1. Rest the forearm comfortably on a table so the wrist lies just at the end of the table (Figure 1).
2. Hold onto a small weight or soup can with your palm down.
3. Slowly rotate your palm upward to a handshake position (Figure 2), then over until your palm is facing up (Figure 3).
4. Slowly rotate your palm back to the starting position.
5. Repeat for a total of 5 times.
6. Perform the exercise with the opposite hand.

Shoulder Raises

EXERCISE IS TO HELP WITH:
Reaching • General Housework Such as Dusting •
Removing Dishes from the Cabinet • Washing Your Hair

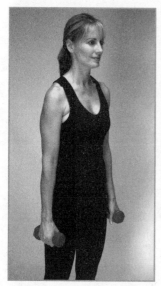

1

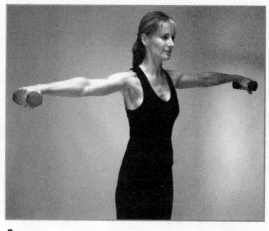

2

1. Start with arms at your side (Figure 1), using a 1- to 3-pound weight (small soup can will also do). Make certain to keep your back straight.
2. Let the weights rest comfortably in your hands.
3. Slowly bring your arms straight out from your side until your arms are at 90 degrees from the floor (Figure 2). Hold this position for a count of 3.
4. Slowly lower your arms to your side.
5. Rest for a count of 3.
6. Repeat this 10 times.

Shoulder Abduction with Wand

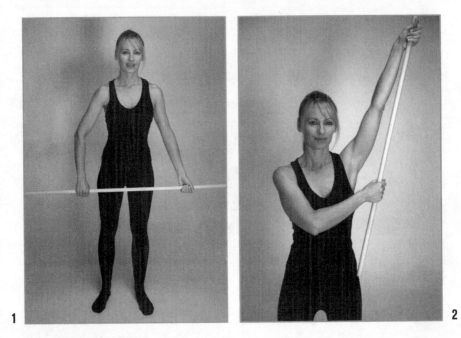

1

2

1. Hold the wand (can use a broomstick) with the palm of your left hand up and the palm of your right hand down (Figure 1).
2. Push the wand directly out from the side of your body until you feel a good stretch (Figure 2).
3. Hold for 3 seconds.
4. Repeat for a total of 5 times. Reverse and perform on the opposite side.

Corner Stretch

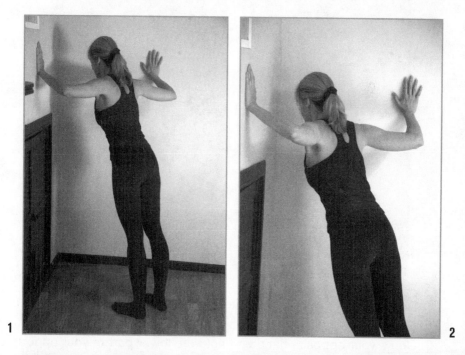

1

2

1. Stand in corner with hands at shoulder level (Figure 1).
2. Keep feet about 3 feet from the corner.
3. Slowly lean forward until a comfortable stretch is felt across the chest (Figure 2).
4. Use your arms to push out to the original starting position.
5. Repeat a total of 5 times.

Biceps Curl

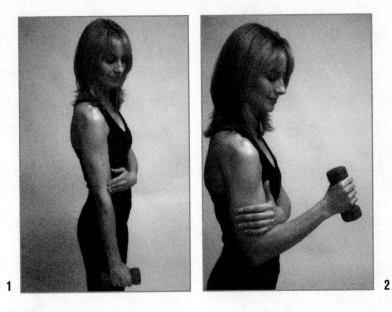

1. Begin with the arm at your side, gently gripping a light weight (Figure 1).
2. Cross your opposite hand and hold the lower part of your upper arm for support.
3. Raise the arm with the weight and hold the position for a count of 3 (Figure 2).
4. Slowly lower the arm to the neutral position.
5. Repeat the exercise 10 times with each arm.

Shoulder Blade Retraction

EXERCISE IS TO HELP WITH:
Shoulder Flexibility • Posture Improvement

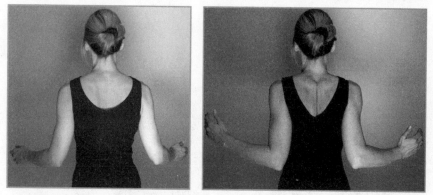

1

2

1. Begin with arms at your side, bent at 90 degrees at the elbow (Figure 1).
2. Pinch your shoulder blades together and rotate your arms out, keeping your elbows bent (Figure 2).
3. Hold this position for three seconds.
4. Slowly relax your shoulder blades and bring your arms forward to the starting position.
5. Repeat for a total of 5 times.

Lower Back Stretch

EXERCISE IS TO HELP WITH:
Lower Back Flexibility • Lower Back Strength •
Getting Out of a Chair • Posture Improvement

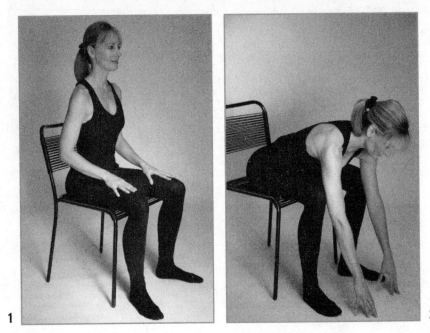

1

2

1. Sit in a chair with your knees spread apart (Figure 1).
2. Bend forward to floor (Figure 2).
3. You should feel a comfortable stretch in your lower back.
4. Hold this position for 3 seconds.
5. Slowly sit up.
6. Perform a total of 5 times.

Back Flexion

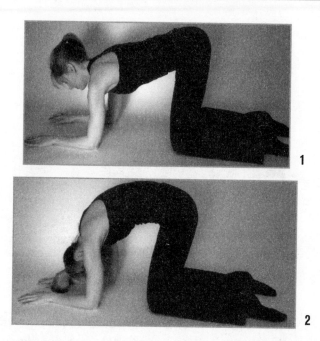

1

2

1. Start on your elbows and knees (neutral position). Position your elbows directly beneath your shoulders and your knees directly beneath your hips. Gaze at the floor (Figure 1).
2. When you are ready to begin, breathe in deeply. Gently pull the abdominal muscles backward toward the spine, tucking the tailbone (coccyx) down and under and gently contracting the buttocks. Press firmly downward with your hands in order to stay lifted off of the shoulders, and press the middle of your back toward the ceiling, rounding your spine upward. Curl your head inward (Figure 2).
3. Hold this position for a count of 5, and then relax.
4. Repeat 4 more times.

* USE A PILLOW UNDER YOUR KNEES FOR MORE COMFORT

Back Extension

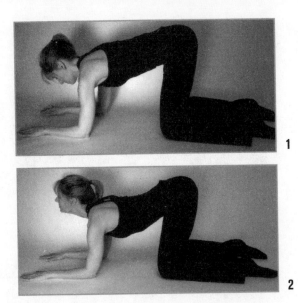

1

2

1. Start on your elbows and knees (neutral position). Position your elbows directly beneath your shoulders and your knees directly beneath the hips. Make your back horizontal and flat. Gaze at the floor (Figure 1).
2. As you inhale, release the grip of the buttocks, reversing the tilt of your pelvis, and curving your spine into a smoothly arched back-bend. Continue pressing downward with your hands to lengthen the arms and stay lifted off of the shoulders. Lift your chest away from the waist, lift your head up, slide the shoulder blades down your back (Figure 2).
3. Hold this position for a count of 5, relax.
4. Repeat 4 more times.

* USE A PILLOW UNDER YOUR KNEES FOR MORE COMFORT

Sitting External Hip Rotation

EXERCISE IS TO HELP WITH:
Overall Flexibility • Walking • Turning While Walking

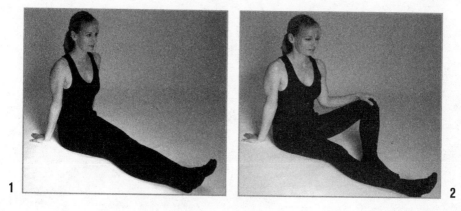

1. Begin seated on the floor, legs in front, using your arms for support (Figure 1).
2. Gradually move your left foot along your right leg until your left foot is even with your right knee. Point your left knee to the left (Figure 2).
3. Hold this position for a count of 5.
4. Gradually slide your left foot down to the starting position.
5. Repeat 4 more times.
6. Repeat for the right hip.

Sitting Internal Hip Rotation

EXERCISE IS TO HELP WITH:
Overall Flexibility • Walking • Turning While Walking • Playing Sports

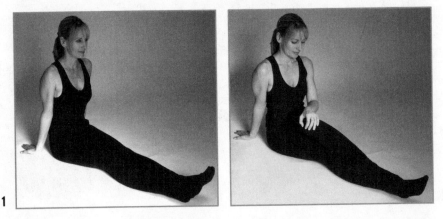

1

2

1. Begin seated on the floor, legs in front, using your arms for support (Figure 1).
2. Gradually move your left foot along your right leg until your left foot is even with the right knee. Point your left knee toward your right leg (Figure 2).
3. Hold this position for a count of 5.
4. Gradually slide your left foot down to the starting position.
5. Repeat 4 more times.
6. Repeat for the right hip.

Sitting Hip Abduction

EXERCISE IS TO HELP WITH:
Overall Flexibility • Walking

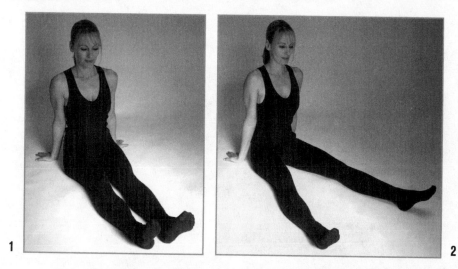

1

2

1. Begin seated on the floor, legs in front and feet together. Use your arms for support (Figure 1).
2. Keep the right leg in front, aligned with the right shoulder. Raise the left leg slightly off the floor and move it toward the left as far as you can (Figure 2). Rest.
3. Raise the left leg slightly off the floor and bring it back to the neutral position.
4. Repeat 4 more times.
5. Repeat exercise for the right leg.

Hip Flexion

EXERCISE IS TO HELP WITH:
Improving Posture • Increasing Flexiblity • Picking Up Light Objects

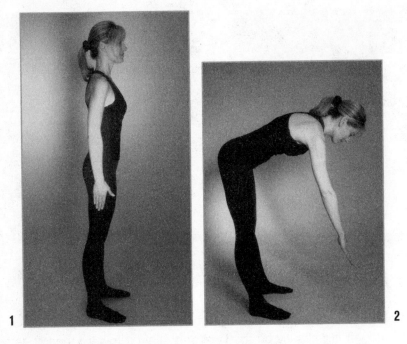

1   2

1. Start standing straight with your arms at your side (Figure 1).
2. Bend at the waist, keeping your legs straight. Relax and let your
   upper body hang down in front of you (Figure 2). Do not force
   your body down. There is no need to touch your toes.
3. Hold this position for 5 seconds.
4. Slowly raise your upper body back to the original position. Hold
   for 3 seconds and repeat.
5. Perform this for a total of 10 repetitions.

Standing Hip Abduction

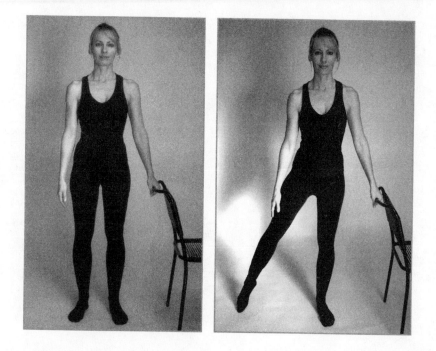

1. Use a chair for support, holding it with your left hand. Put your weight on your left leg (Figure 1).
2. Begin with feet 4 inches apart. Carefully and slowly move your right leg out to the side (Figure 2).
3. Hold this position for a count of 3, and then slowly lower your right foot to the floor. Return to the original position.
4. Repeat this exercise another 4 times.
5. Rest, reverse position, and perform exercise for left leg.

Standing Hip Extension

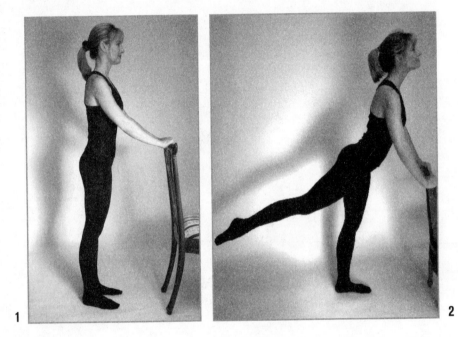

1. Use a chair for support, holding it with both hands (Figure 1).
2. Put your weight on your left leg. Extend your right leg as far as you can. Keep your toe pointed out (Figure 2). If you have back problems, only bring your leg out 3 inches.
3. Hold this position for a count of 3.
4. Take 3 seconds to lower your leg, returning to the original position.
5. Repeat exercise a total of 5 times.
6. Rest, then repeat exercise for the left leg.

Standing Hip and Knee Flexion

> **EXERCISE IS TO HELP WITH:**
> Walking • Getting Up from a Chair •
> Walking Up Stairs • Getting In and Out of a Car

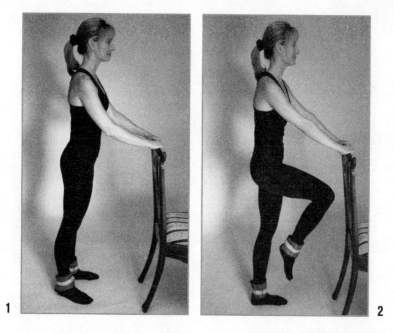

1

2

1. Use a chair for support with both your hands (Figure 1).
2. Put your weight on your left leg. (Ankle weights are optional.)
3. Raise your right leg to 90 degrees, bending at the knee (Figure 2). Take 3 seconds to raise the leg, and then hold it in place for 1 second.
4. Take 3 seconds to lower the leg.
5. Repeat with left leg, alternating legs until you have done 5 repetitions with each leg.

Standing Knee Flexion

EXERCISE IS TO HELP WITH:
Walking • Getting Up From a Chair •
Walking Up Stairs • Getting In and Out of a Car

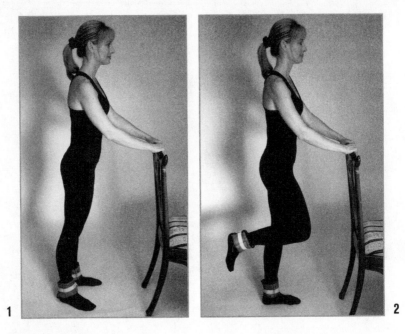

1

2

1. Use a chair for support with both your hands (Figure 1).
2. Put your weight on your left leg. (Ankle weights are optional.) Bend the right knee (Figure 2).
3. Take 3 seconds to raise the leg, and then hold it in place for 1 second.
4. Take 3 seconds to lower the leg, returning to the original position.
5. Repeat with left leg, alternating legs until you have done 5 repetitions with each leg.

Standing Toe Raises

EXERCISE IS TO HELP WITH:
Maintaining Good Posture • Walking • Walking Up Stairs

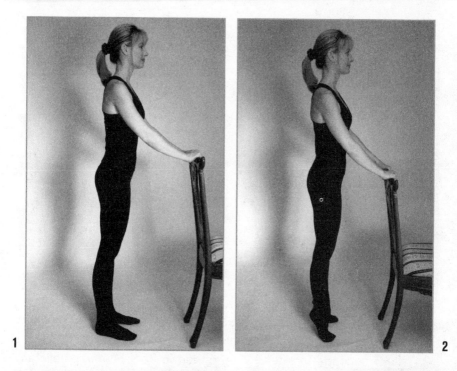

1

2

1. Use a chair for support, holding on with both your hands (Figure 1).
2. Rise up on toes of both feet (Figure 2). Take 3 seconds to rise up on toes, and hold in place for 1 second.
3. Take 3 seconds to lower heels to the ground.

Sitting Knee Extension

EXERCISE IS TO HELP WITH:
Walking • Getting Up From a Chair

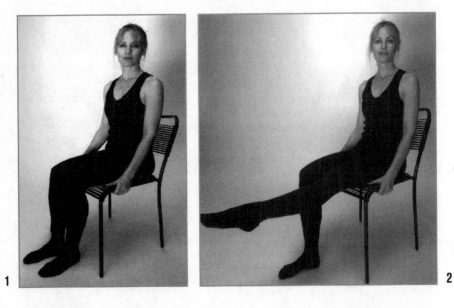

1

2

1. Sit in a chair, with your back resting against the back of the chair.
2. Hold onto the sides of the chair for support (Figure 1).
3. Take 3 seconds to extend your left leg in front of you, parallel to the floor (Figure 2). (Ankle weights are optional and can be used when you are ready.)
4. Hold this position for 1 second, then take 3 seconds to lower your leg to the starting position.
5. Repeat with the right leg.
6. Alternate legs until you have performed 5 repetitions with each leg.

Neck Flexion and Extension

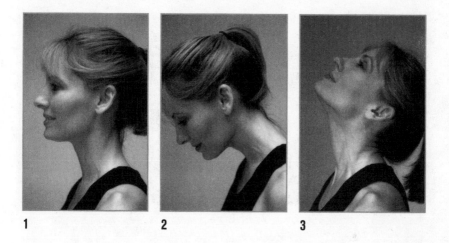

1   2   3

1. Start with your head in a neutral position (Figure 1).
2. Slowly bring your chin towards your chest, hold for 3 seconds (Figure 2).
3. Return to the neutral position for 2 seconds.
4. Bring your chin up to the ceiling, hold for 3 seconds (Figure 3).
5. Repeat for a total of 10 repetitions.

Neck Rotation Exercises

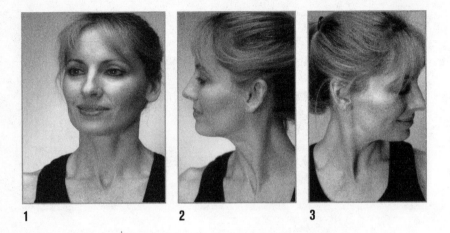

1   2   3

1. Start with your head in a neutral position (Figure 1).
2. Slowly turn your head and look to the right, hold for 3 seconds (Figure 2).
3. Return to the neutral position for 2 seconds.
4. Slowly turn your head and look to the left, hold for 3 seconds (Figure 3).
5. Repeat for a total of 10 repetitions.

Neck Lateral Flexion Exercises

EXERCISE IS TO HELP WITH:
Driving • Combing Your Hair • Drying Your Hair

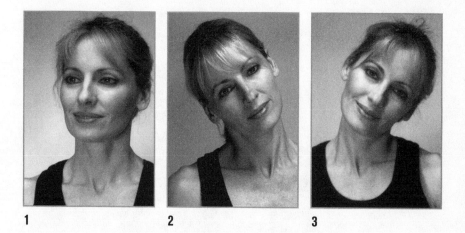

1   2   3

1. Start with your head in a neutral position (Figure 1).
2. Slowly bring your right ear down towards your right shoulder, hold for 3 seconds (Figure 2).
3. Return to the neutral position for 2 seconds.
4. Slowly bring your left ear down towards your left shoulder, hold for 3 seconds (Figure 3).
5. Repeat for a total of 10 repetitions.

Ankle Circles

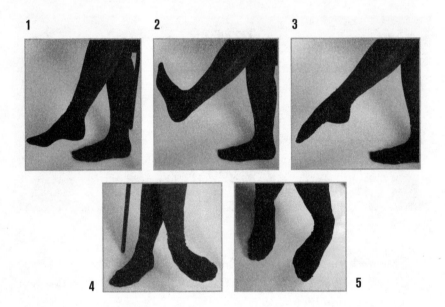

1. Sit in a chair with your right leg comfortably crossed over your left leg (Figure 1).
2. Flex your right foot and hold it for 3 seconds (Figure 2).
3. Point your right foot towards the ground and hold it for 3 seconds (Figure 3).
4. Move your entire ankle to the side away from your body, hold it for 3 seconds (Figure 4).
5. Move your entire ankle to the inside towards your body, hold it for 3 seconds (Figure 5).
6. Repeat for a total of 10 times.
7. Perform exercise on the left ankle.

7
CHAPTER

A Mixed Bag of Miracles and Mundane Medicinals

ARTHRITIS CAN ROB you of your quality of life, your peace of mind, and even your ability to cope with the simple demands of everyday living. Brushing your teeth, opening a door, even getting out of bed in the morning can turn into exercises in pain management. If you're facing these kinds of ordeals from morning until night, day after day, year after year, it would certainly be understandable if you went looking for a miracle. Unfortunately, you're unlikely to find any—although there are plenty of hucksters in the world willing to sell you a counterfeit.

Now, I don't mean to imply that miracles never happen. In medicine, we see them all the time. People with advanced cancers go into remission. Patients on the verge of death suddenly recover. Predictions that someone will never walk again dissolve into memory as he/she crosses the finish line in a marathon. There is no doubt that these events occur all the time—although we don't really know why, and they tend to happen with seemingly complete unpredictability. What we do know is that miracles don't usually occur as a result of some untested gimmick or service purchased over the Internet or provided at an island resort in the Caribbean. In other words, the hucksters don't have them.

But while there may not be any real "miracle cures" for arthritis, there are some things you can do beyond diet, supplements, exercise, and medication that can help you ease your pain. The trick is to learn what can actually help and what is pure quackery. Start with the list below.

Bee Sting Therapy

Products manufactured by honey bees, including both honey and venom, have been used medicinally throughout recorded history. Hippocrates, the 'father of medicine,' used bee stings to treat arthritic joint pain over two thousand years ago. The entry of *apitherapy*, as it's called, into modern medicine began when an Australian physician named Phillip Terc published an article on the subject in 1888.

Today, many people believe that bee venom can be used to treat both RA and multiple sclerosis (MS). In fact, there was enough interest in the subject to motivate researchers at Georgetown University, in Washington, D.C., to do a trial study of its effect on MS patients. The purpose of the study was to establish the safety of injecting very low doses of bee venom extract into patients. The study looked at too few people to come to any firm conclusions about the medicinal effectiveness of the venom, but although the researchers found the extract safe to use, they do *not* recommend injection of raw venom through live bee stings. Bees don't control dosage, and there is a very real danger of allergic reaction that could result in death.

There is actually some logic to the idea that bee venom could be used to treat arthritis, as it contains several anti-inflammatory chemicals. One, called *melitin*, is a hundred times more potent than cortisone. Another, called *adolapin*, also blocks pain. However, the place to study the effects of these substances is in controlled clinical trials, where doctors can carefully monitor patients' side effects and reactions—NOT in the kitchen (or office) of some shaman who stings you with live bees.

In any case, it would be difficult to find anyone willing to administer apitherapy these days. After a few bad allergic reactions and some consequent deaths, the FDA started cracking down on the practice.

MAKING LIFE A LITTLE EASIER

If you have limited hand function, hard rubber doorknob extenders convert a round doorknob into an "easy grab" lever for extra leverage. They are easy to install (they usually slip over your current doorknob) and are available at many hardware stores and surgical supplies stores. You can also look online for rehab equipment and supplies.

Chiropractic

Chiropractic was first developed in 1895 by Daniel David Palmer, a colorful character who had in the course of his life been a beekeeper, a school teacher, a grocery store owner, and a practitioner of various branches of alternative medicine. One of Palmer's patients was a deaf janitor who had a lump on his spine. Palmer believed that a connection existed between the lump and the deafness, so he began manipulating his patient's spine until the lump disappeared. He later reported that the patient's deafness then went away as well.

This led to the fundamental theory of chiropractic: The body is built to heal itself, but to do that successfully, there must be clear signaling between its control center, the brain, and the rest of its organs. To get to and from the brain, these signals must travel through the spinal cord. If there is a kink in the spinal cord, the signals become distorted, weakened, or blocked—just like water building up behind a kink in a hose—and proper healing can't take place. In chiropractic theory, these kinks happen as a result of slight misalignments, called *subluxations,* of the vertebrae in the spine, and manipulating them back into place can help cure disease.

Not all modern chiropractors agree with the subluxation theory. In fact, some have openly criticized it and refuse to do manipulation to cure any condition but back pain unrelated to any disease. In 1997, the

American Medical Association, long antagonistic toward chiropractic, did concede finally that ". . . manipulation has been shown to have a reasonably good degree of efficacy in ameliorating back pain, headache, and similar musculoskeletal complaints." So finally, a small group of chiropractors and conventional doctors may be discovering some small area of common ground.

That ground is precisely where I think chiropractic can be helpful to OA patients, who very often have back pain. I do not, however, believe that it works by correcting subluxations. It's more likely that the treatments, which can include galvanic nerve stimulation (running a very low electric current through the nerves), massage, and ultrasound, trigger an endorphin release in the brain. Endorphins are powerful pain-blocking chemicals that the body produces on its own. Chiropractic treatments can also cause relaxation, which leads to a reduction of stress on ligaments, and thus, less pain.

The bottom line about chiropractic is that it will not cure your disease, but it may help somewhat with pain control, especially in the back. One

THE MANY FACES OF ARTHRITIS: ANKYLOSING SPONDYLITIS

Ankylosing spondylitis is RA of the spine and sacroiliac joints. Its inflammation can also occur in other organs such as the eyes, lungs, and heart valves. It most often develops in adolescent and young adult males, although it can strike at any age, and Native Americans are more prone to it than other racial groups. It can trigger back pain that comes and goes or it can develop into a chronic, progressively severe condition that ends up causing loss of motion and deformity. Treatment, which consists of non-steroidal anti-inflammatory drugs along with rehabilitation therapy, can be very successful, especially if the disease is caught early. Medications such as methotrexate and the newer biologics (Humira, Enbrel, Remicade) have been successfully used in the treatment of ankylosing spondylitis.

caveat: I would not recommend spinal manipulation for RA patients, who often have significant back and neck issues. It might aggravate existing problems. Massage, ultrasound, and galvanic stimulation, however, should all be quite safe.

Homeopathy

Like chiropractic, homeopathy is a branch of alternative medicine. It started with a medical doctor, Samuel Hahnemann, who began experimenting with homeopathic remedies in 1790. The theory behind the practice is that ingesting appropriate substances (extracted from plants, minerals, or animals) in extremely dilute amounts will stimulate the body to mount immune defenses against particular diseases.

The remedies are supposed to cause the same symptoms in healthy people as those they're supposed to treat in sick patients—"like cures like," as the saying goes. Hahnemann got the idea when he experimented with a South American tree bark that was used to treat malaria. When he ingested the bark himself, he developed symptoms that were very much like those of the disease.

I have not been convinced by homeopathy. Laboratory analysis of some remedies has shown them to be so dilute that they have no trace of active substance left in them. They're pure water. It's sort of like mixing a dry martini by just passing the cap of the vermouth bottle over the gin like a magic wand. It's as if you don't need the vermouth, just its "essence," which mystically turns gin or vodka into "martini." Frankly, it's nonsense—whether we're talking about bartending or homeopathy. Furthermore, I'm not aware of any scientific studies that show that homeopathic treatments have helped with either RA or OA.

So now you may be thinking, *if homeopathy is so ineffective, how did it become so popular?* And why did our grandparents and great grandparents have such faith in it?

Frankly, a couple of hundred years ago, allopathic (conventional) doctors were more likely to kill a patient than cure him. Our therapies included purging, bloodletting, and dosing with toxic chemicals like mercury. When our patients got better, they did so in spite of our help, not because of it. Homeopaths, on the other hand, didn't kill anyone, and their patients often got better—because if you don't interfere with a body's healing, it might very well recover on its own. So there was a place and time when homeopathic medicine may have made some sort of sense. It kept the dangerous allopaths away, and it did no harm. Today, however, modern medicine has come a very long way, and we do have safe and effective ways to treat chronic diseases like arthritis.

By the way, homeopathic remedies should not be confused with herbal medicines. Many herbs are chemically active in the body, and some can actually be used to improve health or treat disease. Others can be quite harmful.

Hypnosis

Hypnosis describes a "trance" state, similar to daydreaming. When you're hypnotized, you're both more focused and more open to suggestion than when you're in a normal waking state. The use of hypnosis in medicine extends back to antiquity, but the term was first coined in 1842 by James Braid, who experimented with trance states to cure organic disease. He didn't have much luck. But other physicians of the time had long reported using trance states to perform painless surgeries.

As Braid found out the hard way, hypnosis is not going to cure anybody's disease, but it can be very good for pain control—as can other mind/body techniques such as transcendental meditation and biofeedback. Unfortunately, hypnosis doesn't work for everybody. Some people are simply less hypnotizable than others, and among those who can be

MAKING LIFE A LITTLE EASIER

Foam hair rollers make great cushy grips. Slide off the foam tubes. Slide the foam onto pens, pencils, forks, spoons, or any small object that is hard to hold.

hypnotized, some can't attain more than the most superficial level of trance. Still, if there is somebody who does not have a serious inflammatory process and is experiencing mild to moderate discomfort, it's not unreasonable to give hypnosis a try.

Ultrasound

Ultrasound treatment is a perfectly legitimate therapy used by many physical therapists. Again, it will not cure your arthritis, but the extremely high and low sound waves (outside of the normal hearing range) generated by an ultrasound machine will penetrate your muscles and cause them to grow warm. The warmth causes tissues to relax, reducing muscle tension and spasms, and therefore, pain. The rise in muscle temperature can also cause blood vessels to dilate, promoting increased circulation to the area. At the right frequencies, sound waves can even reduce inflammation. You can buy portable ultrasound therapy machines for about $200 on the Internet, but I would rather you not perform procedures on yourself without the supervision of a healthcare professional.

Along with ultrasound, many physical therapists and occupational therapists today use *phonophoresis* and *iontophoresis* to help control pain and inflammation. Phonophoresis uses high frequency sound waves to drive molecules of medication through the skin and into inflamed or painful areas. Iontophoresis does the same thing, but uses an electric current instead of sound to carry the medication where it has to go. Both techniques are safe and effective.

Acupuncture

Acupuncture was first used in China about 2,000 years ago. Traditional theory states that our bodies contain a basic life energy called Qi, and this energy flows along lines called *meridians,* which are located just under the skin. If the flow of Qi is hindered in any way, the body goes out of balance and illness occurs. Disorders in every part of the body are represented by acupuncture points, which are said to be spots where meridians come to the surface of the skin. Stimulating these points with very small, slender needles corrects energy flow and restores health.

Most legitimate modern practitioners admit that acupuncture doesn't actually cure disease, and the Qi theory can't be tested or proven through scientific study. Nevertheless, the procedure does seem to work, and in my experience, is fairly effective for managing pain. More credible than the Qi theory, I think, is the idea that acupuncture needles stimulate nerve centers and trigger endorphin release, which blocks pain. My patients have also had good experience with acupressure, which means simply applying some gentle pressure, with a finger to acupuncture points, rather than inserting a needle.

Psychotherapy

Some folks believe that the body/mind connection is so strong that you can cure arthritis in the body by healing the mind. For a while, a similar fad raged around cancer treatment. I'm not convinced that it's possible. However, I do believe that keeping a healthy emotional and mental state is extremely important in arthritis treatment. Although we don't usually think of the brain as an organ of the immune system, it is in fact a very important part of that system. It can, for example, express either pro- or anti-inflammatory neurotransmitters, and your state of mind can affect which it will choose.

If you recall, back in the 1970s political journalist Norman Cousins developed a form of extremely painful spinal arthritis called *ankylosing spondylitis*. As he grappled with the disease, he came to discover that a big belly laugh could relieve his pain for up to two hours at a time. It turned out that for him, watching Marx Brothers films was more healing than any medicine he could buy.

As it turns out, investigators discovered that laughter causes the brain to release anti-inflammatory proteins. Further studies have shown that people who think sad thoughts develop more inflammation than people who generally think happy ones.

So for patients who are depressed, it may pay off to see a psychotherapist, or even a psychiatrist who can prescribe antidepressant drugs.

DEPRESSION AND RA

At least 20 percent of all patients with RA become seriously depressed. There are many reasons for this. Part of it simply has to do with the disease's effect on brain chemistry. But there's also the fact that when you can't even turn a doorknob, you can easily begin to feel frustrated and hopeless. Unfortunately, that can play havoc with arthritis treatment. I see it again and again in my practice. Unless patients deal with their depression, their arthritis simply doesn't get better. Once they go into treatment for the depression, however, it's amazing how much better their arthritis becomes. Within six weeks of going on an antidepressant, many experience significant improvement in their joint pain, they're more able to cope with activities of daily living, and even their blood tests improve.

Massage

Massage is probably the oldest form of medical healing we know of. It's depicted on the walls of ancient Egyptian tombs, and the Chinese were writing about it nearly 3,000 years ago. Modern Swedish massage was invented by a doctor named Per Henrick Ling. He designed his system around the principles of gymnastic movements and borrowed techniques from many other systems, including some from the Far East and many from the classical world of Egypt, Greece, and Rome. It's currently used in many medical settings, from drug treatment programs to cancer clinics, but can it help with arthritis?

Hippocrates wrote in the 5th century B. C. that ". . . rubbing can bind a joint that is too loose, and loosen a joint that is too rigid." I don't know if he was talking specifically about arthritis, but he well could have been. Massage therapy is great for your joints if done properly. It works on many different levels. It stimulates endorphin release, it relaxes the muscles around the joint, and it increases blood flow around the joint.

THE MAGIC OF MAGNETS AND COPPER JEWELRY

About fifteen years ago, people began buying machines that purported to improve circulation to the joints by exposing them to magnetic fields. At about the same time, people were buying copper bracelets to relieve their joint pain—actually a resurgence of an old folk remedy. The theory behind the bracelets was that your skin would absorb copper from them, which could cure, or at least relieve the pain of OA and RA. If you do a search on these remedies on the Web, you may read that their efficacy is "still in question" or "yet unproven." It's time to set the record straight. There is nothing about either "cure" that is still in question. Both are snake oil, worthless quackery.

DMSO

DMSO, short for *dimethyl sulfoxide,* is an industrial solvent produced as a by-product in the paper pulp industry. At solutions between 70 and 90 percent, it easily penetrates human skin and also has the ability to carry certain drugs with it. Some studies have shown it to be a powerful antioxidant, anti-inflammatory, and pain reliever. All kinds of claims have been made for its efficacy in treating a number of conditions, including RA. There are two fundamental issues with DMSO use. The first is that we don't need DMSO. These days we have treatments for arthritis that are far more effective and that are just as safe to use. The second problem is aesthetic. It can give you bad breath and body odor. During some trials of the substance, the unpleasant scent was so powerful that subjects had to move into separate bedrooms away from their spouses.

When the body processes DMSO, various by-products, called *metabolites* are produced. One of these, MSM (methylsulphonylmethane) has turned out to have many of the same medicinal properties as DMSO, but doesn't cause any odiferous side effects, and it has been approved by the FDA for at least one medical condition: cystitis. Of the two substances, I would recommend MSM. It seems to have almost no toxicity, and many people take it as nutritional supplement to control pain and inflammation. You can purchase it at your local health food store, or from various websites that offer vitamins and herbal supplements.

Special Diets

And then there were those special, often bizarre eating plans that were supposed to cure joint pain—like the sauerkraut and honey diet, or gin and raisins diet. For the latter, you're supposed to soak the raisins for two weeks and then eat them. For pain relief, you'd probably do better just to throw out the raisins and drink the gin.

If you want a diet that can actually reduce inflammation and arthritis pain, help you lose weight, and possibly even bring your cholesterol under control, try the one offered in the next chapter.

CHAPTER

Putting It All Together

So NOW LET'S put everything into one package: The Arthritis Doctor's 28-Day Program, which uses supplements, exercise, and diet to help your body reduce inflammation, maintain your range of motion, and decrease mild to moderate arthritic pain.

What is mild to moderate? In the first chapter, you took a brief quiz called the ADQ and calculated a score between 0 and 24. If your score is between 0 and 8, you probably have mild, early-stage arthritis and should be able to handle it with exercise and supplements alone. Here again are the exercises and supplements that will help most.

The Arthritis Doctor's Superset

The ten exercises below should be done five or six days a week as part of your Arthritis Doctor's 28-Day Program. Do one set of ten repetitions for each exercise the first week. Add another set for the second week, and yet another for the third, making a total of three sets (thirty repetitions) for each exercise. On week four, add in twenty minutes of walking, three days a week.

1. **Pip Finger Flexion** (Page 74)
   This exercise will help with grasping, writing, and holding onto eating utensils.

2. **Wrist Flexion** (Page 77)

   This exercise will help with dressing, cooking, eating, and personal hygiene.

3. **Elbow Turns** (Page 80)

   This exercise will help with turning a doorknob and turning a key.

4. **Shoulder Abduction with Wand** (Page 82)

   This exercise will help with reaching, general housework such as dusting, and removing dishes from the cabinet.

5. **Corner Stretch** (Page 83)

   This exercise will help with overall flexibility, increasing shoulder flexibility, increasing wrist flexibility, and increasing shoulder blade flexibility.

6. **Lower Back Stretch** (Page 86)

   This exercise will help with lower back flexibility and strength, getting out of a chair, and posture improvement.

7. **Standing Hip and Knee Flexion** (Page 95)

   This exercise will help with pivoting and reaching to the side.

8. **Standing Toe Raises** (Page 97)

   This exercise will help with maintaining good posture, walking, and climbing stairs.

9. **Neck Flexion and Extension** (Page 99)

   This exercise will help with driving, watching movies, and nodding your head "yes."

10. **Neck Rotation Exercises** (Page 100)

    This exercise will help with driving, kissing, and shaking your head "no."

The Arthritis Doctor's Super Supplements

The 28-day plan's supplements are easy. There are only three: calcium, vitamin D, and omega–3 fatty acids (fish oil or flax). Here are the dosages and precautions:

Calcium. 1500 to 2000 mg a day. Dosage includes supplements and calcium from other sources, so if you're a big milk drinker, adjust your supplemental dosage accordingly. By the way, there are 306 mg of calcium in a cup of skim milk. Eight ounces of low-fat, plain yogurt contains 415 mg, while the same amount of whole milk yogurt contains 275 mg. Collard greens are very high in calcium. One cup contains 357 mg of calcium. And if you're eating a lot of salmon (which you should be doing), 3 oz contains 181 mg of calcium.

Precautions: Supplemental calcium can cause gas, flatulence, constipation, and bloating. If taken without food, it may cause kidney stones to form.

Vitamin D. 400 IU to 800 IU a day. Vitamin D helps you absorb calcium. The amount you need every day depends on where you live, because exposure to ultraviolet rays from the sun actually cause the body to produce its own vitamin D. If you live in a warm climate in the Southern United States with lots of sun exposure, you'll need only 400 IU (International Units) of vitamin D in supplement form a day. If you live in northern parts of the country where there is less sunlight in the winter (as in the Northeast) or a lot of cloud cover (as in the Northwest), you'll need 800 IU a day. Be aware that milk is often fortified with vitamin D, so if you're a big milk drinker, you may not need to supplement at all.

Precautions: Vitamin D is stored in body fat, and if you take too much it can be toxic. Adults shouldn't exceed 20,000 IU a day, and children shouldn't exceed 2,000 IU a day.

Omega-3 fatty acids. 2000 mg to 3000 mg. You'll need to be a little careful about these supplements when choosing what to take. If you're taking fish oil capsules, the label will most likely list the amount of *fish oil* in one *serving.* You want to know how much *omega-3 fatty acids* are in each capsule. That means you should add up the amounts of eicosapentaenoic acid (EPA) and docosahexaenoic acid (DHA) in each serving, and presuming one serving equals two capsules, you then need to divide that number by two. Complicated, right? It's much easier to take two teaspoons of Carlson's lemon-flavored fish oil every day. It tastes good and doesn't require a lot of math to figure out. Also, if you're taking capsules, make sure the label says "mercury free."

You can supplement with flax instead of fish oil, but because it contains a different kind of omega-3 fatty acid (alpha linolenic acid), you have to take more of it. Whether you're taking it in oil form or adding it to food in meal form, you'll need two tablespoons a day.

Precautions: If you are on any other medication, including aspirin or blood thinners, be sure to let your doctor know that you're taking omega-3 supplements. Combining omega-3s with certain medicines can slightly raise your risk of internal bleeding. Also, if you've had more than 3 oz of wild salmon on any given day, you won't need to take a supplement on that day.

The Arthritis Doctor's 28-Day Super Menu

It's hard to find a bright side to having arthritis, but if there is one, it's this: You get to eat like royalty. Included below are eighty-four delicious meals—that's three a day for twenty-eight days. The ingredients have been carefully selected not only for their wonderful flavors, but also for their healthful, anti-inflammatory properties. Every meal has a high omega-3 content, a low omega-6 content, and an omega-6 to omega-3 ratio below 5 (important for reducing inflammation). Also, each food chosen has a low glycemic index, a low glycemic load, and is low in sodium and cholesterol. And every meal takes only thirty minutes or less to prepare. You'll find recipes for all the dishes in the next chapter.

Remember that it's okay to add in restricted ingredients like sugar or milk on the very rare occasion. If you completely ban foods that you love from your meals, you won't be a happy camper, and you probably won't maintain your diet for long. Just don't allow inflammatory things onto your plate on a regular basis.

You may be surprised that the diet actually includes wine and chocolate. Recent research has shown that both of these foods can, in moderation, be *beneficial* to your health.

Red wine contains an estrogen-like substance called *resveratrol,* which grapes produce naturally to fight off fungus. Not only has resveratrol been shown to reduce heart disease among wine drinkers, but in high amounts (more than you can get in wine), it may reduce most or all of the diseases associated with aging—heart disease, cancer, diabetes, etc. Of course, you don't want too much alcohol in your diet (and none at all if you have a problem with drinking). American doctors recommend no more than two five-ounce glasses a day for men and one for women. Interestingly, Italian researchers recommend twice those amounts.

Dark chocolate with at least a 70 percent cocoa content contains significant amounts of *flavonoids,* substances that help protect the body from the damaging effects of free radicals, and thus inflammation. Milk chocolate does not have similarly high amounts of flavonoids, so unfortunately, it is *not* part of the Super Diet. The good news is that chocolate is not as high in bad fats as we once thought. About a third of the fat is *oleic acid,* a monosaturated fat like olive oil that may be healthful to your heart. Another third is *stearic acid,* which is a saturated fat but has been shown not to raise cholesterol levels in the bloodstream. The remaining third is *palmitic acid,* which is not a healthful fat and does raise levels of HDL. So chocolate is allowed, but again, a small amount—a piece or two—now and then.

A note about weight loss: You can use this diet to lose weight, gain weight, or maintain your current weight. The meals in the 28-day sample menu contain about 1,500 calories each. That's enough to maintain a weight of about 135 lbs. If your current weight is higher and you follow the diet exactly as given, you'll gradually shed pounds.

Below are some guidelines to use in adjusting the menu to fit your own goals with regard to your weight. Simply increase or decrease the portion size of anti-inflammatory foods to bring your meals into the calorie range you need.

To Lose Weight:

Divide your body weight in pounds by 2.2. This gives you your body weight in kilograms. Multiply that number by 15. Multiply the same number by 20. The two final numbers represent the range of calories you need every day to lose weight healthfully. Here's an example, using a person—let's call her Kathy—who weighs 176 pounds.

176/2.2 = 80 kilograms

80 x 15 = 1,200 calories

80 x 20 = 1,600 calories

If Kathy wants to lose weight, she should eat anywhere from 1,200 to 1,600 calories a day. Once she reaches her weight gain goal, she will need to calculate her calorie range to maintain that weight. By the way, technically, a calorie is actually called a *kilocalorie*. That's why you'll sometimes see the abbreviation "Kcal" used.

To Maintain Weight:

If Kathy wants to keep her weight right where it is, she should divide her body weight in pounds by 2.2 to get her weight in kilograms, then multiply that number by 20 and again the same number by 25. The two final numbers represent the range of calories she'll need every day to maintain her weight. Here's how it works out:

176/2.2 = 80 kilograms

80 x 20 = 1,600 calories

80 x 25 = 2,000 calories

So Kathy's calorie range to maintain her weight is 1,600 to 2,000 calories a day.

To Gain Weight:

Finally, if Kathy wants to gain some weight, she should divide her body weight in pounds by 2.2 to get her weight in kilograms, then multiply that number by 25 and again the same number by 30. The two final numbers represent the range of calories she'll need every day to maintain her weight. Here's how it works out:

176/2.2 = 80 kilograms

80 x 25 = 2,000 calories

80 x 30 = 2,400 calories

So Kathy's calorie range to gain weight is 2,000 to 2,400 calories a day. Once she reaches her weight gain goal, she will need to calculate her calorie range to maintain that weight.

The Arthritis Doctor's 28-Day Meal Plan

Following on pages 122–149 is the 28-Day Meal Plan. A number next to a meal or snack indicates the page on which you may find the recipe. Most menu choices in the 28-Day Meal Plan are among the recipes included on pages 151–201.

Breakfast

V-8 Calcium Enriched Vegetable Juice (8 Oz) (1 Serving)
Omega Oatmeal (1 Serving)—p. 177

Lunch

Ginger Tuna Salad (1 Serving)—p. 168
Carrots (1/2 Cup)
Celery (1/2 Cup)
Whole Wheat Pita Bread (1 Ea)

Dinner

Chopped Salad with Special Balsamic Vinaigrette Dressing
    (1 Serving)—p. 161
Three Spice Baked Chicken (1 Serving)—p. 195
Brown Rice with Turmeric (1 Serving)—p. 157
Broccoli and Garlic (1 Serving)—p. 157

Evening Snack

Stonyfield Farm Vanilla Nonfat Frozen Yogurt (1 Serving)
Raspberries (1/4 Cup)

Nutritional Information Day Total

Amount Per Serving	
Calories	1570.82
Calories From Fat (29%)	449.92
	% Daily Value
Total Fat 52.85g	**81%**
Saturated Fat 6.99g	**35%**
Cholesterol 111.56mg	**37%**
Sodium 1245.02mg	**52%**
Potassium 3809.24mg	**109%**
Carbohydrates 206.54g	**69%**
Dietary Fiber 39.12g	**156%**
Sugar 46.89g	
Sugar Alcohols 0.00g	
Net Carbohydrates 167.42g	
Protein 85.55g	**171%**

For a nutritional chart for each
meal, see Appendix A, p. 226.

Breakfast

Power Tomato Juice (1 Serving)—p. 180
Harriet's Homemade Granola (1 Serving)—p. 170
Nonfat Milk (1/2 Cup)
Blueberries (1/4 Cup)

Lunch

Tropical Fruit Salad (1 Serving)—p. 196
Chicken Pita Sandwich (1 Serving)—p. 160

Dinner

Grapefruit (1/2 Fruit (3–3/4" Diameter))
Mustard Salmon (1 Serving)—p. 177
Roasted Asparagus (1 Serving)—p. 181
Long-Grain Brown Rice (1/2 Cup)

Evening Snack

Chocolate Covered Strawberries (1 Serving)—p. 161

Nutritional Information Day Total

Amount Per Serving		
Calories	1581.01	
Calories From Fat (31%)	492.11	
		% Daily Value
Total Fat 56.11g		86%
Saturated Fat 10.44g		52%
Cholesterol 84.42mg		28%
Sodium 976.82mg		41%
Potassium 3097.69mg		89%
Carbohydrates 226.71g		76%
Dietary Fiber 30.91g		124%
Sugar 117.51g		
Sugar Alcohols 0.00g		
Net Carbohydrates 195.80g		
Protein 59.75g		120%

For a nutritional chart for each meal, see Appendix A, p. 227.

Breakfast

Black Cherry Juice (1 Cup)
Veggie Frittata (1 Serving)—p. 198

Lunch

Greek Salad (1 Serving)—p. 168
Hummus (1 Serving)—p. 171
Carrots (1/2 X 1 Cup Strips or Slices)
Celery (1/2 Cup)

Dinner

Bob's Sliced Tomatoes and Onion (1 Serving)—p. 155
Portabella Mushrooms Stuffed with Crab (1 Serving)—p. 179
Peas (1 Cup)
Melons, Cantaloupe, Fresh (1/2 Ea)

Evening Snack

Ricotta and Blueberry Parfaits (1 Serving)—p. 181

Nutritional Information Day Total

Amount Per Serving		
Calories	1534.77	
Calories From Fat (31%)	474.24	
		% Daily Value
Total Fat 54.36g		**84%**
Saturated Fat 17.62g		**88%**
Cholesterol 196.86mg		**66%**
Sodium 1780.28mg		**74%**
Potassium 6016.08mg		**172%**
Carbohydrates 192.34g		**64%**
Dietary Fiber 32.20g		**129%**
Sugar 103.59g		
Sugar Alcohols 0.00g		
Net Carbohydrates 160.14g		
Protein 86.26g		**173%**

For a nutritional chart for each
meal, see Appendix A, p. 228.

Breakfast

Omega Oatmeal (1 Serving)—p. 177
Nonfat Plain Yogurt (1 Cup)
Blueberries (1/2 Cup)

Lunch

Brandon's Black Bean Salsa (1 Serving)—p. 156
Avocado Pita Sandwich (1 Serving)—p. 153

Dinner

Tossed Salad with Special Balsamic Vinaigrette Dressing
(1 Serving)—p. 196
Garlic Shrimp in White Wine over Whole Wheat Linguini
(1 Serving)—p. 165
Green Snap Beans (1/2 Cup)

Evening Snack

Sliced Peaches with Raspberry, Pomegranate, and Ginger
Topping (1 Serving)—p. 189

DAY 4

Nutritional Information Day Total

Amount Per Serving		
Calories		1524.00
Calories From Fat (31%)		473.30
		% Daily Value
Total Fat 54.84g		**84%**
Saturated Fat 8.34g		**42%**
Cholesterol 222.13mg		**74%**
Sodium 1176.16mg		**49%**
Potassium 3490.31mg		**100%**
Carbohydrates 201.48g		**67%**
Dietary Fiber 41.03g		**164%**
Sugar 36.42g		
Sugar Alcohols 0.00g		
Net Carbohydrates 160.45g		
Protein 69.46g		**139%**

For a nutritional chart for each
meal, see Appendix A, p. 229.

Breakfast

Margaux's Mango and Banana Smoothie (1 Serving)—p. 174

Scrambled Eggs with Onions, Green Peppers (1 Serving)—
p. 185

Toasted Whole Wheat Bread (1 Slice)

Lunch

Gazpacho (1 Serving)—p. 166

Grilled Island Shrimp Wrap (1 Serving)—p. 169

Dinner

Macadamia Nut Encrusted Mahi-Mahi (1 Serving)—p. 173

Brown Rice with Turmeric (1/2 Serving)—p. 157

Yellow Squash with Lemon (1 Serving)—p. 200

Cantaloupe, Fresh (1 Wedge)

Evening Snack

Chocolate Covered Strawberries (1 Serving)—p. 161

DAY 5

Nutritional Information Day Total

Amount Per Serving		
Calories	1301.83	
Calories From Fat (49%)	636.25	
		% Daily Value
Total Fat 72.40g		**111%**
Saturated Fat 12.96g		**65%**
Cholesterol 43.56mg		**15%**
Sodium 1184.41mg		**49%**
Potassium 3323.18mg		**95%**
Carbohydrates 119.80g		**40%**
Dietary Fiber 18.74g		**75%**
Sugar 57.07g		
Sugar Alcohols 0.00g		
Net Carbohydrates 101.06g		
Protein 52.92g		**106%**

For a nutritional chart for each
meal, see Appendix A, p. 230.

Breakfast

Mixed Berries with Yogurt and Almonds (1 Serving)—p. 176
Toasted Whole Wheat English Muffins (1 Ea)
Fat Free Cream Cheese (1 Oz)

Lunch

Black Cherry Juice (1 Cup)
Chopped Salad with Special Balsamic Vinaigrette Dressing
    (1 Serving)—p. 161
Whole Wheat Bread (1 Slice)

Dinner

Sweet Potato and Leek Soup (1 Serving)—p. 193
London Broil with Garlic Marinade (1 Serving)—p. 172
Horseradish Sauce (1 Serving)—p. 171
Feta and Kalamata Puree (1 Serving)—p. 164
Brown Rice with Turmeric (1 Serving)—p. 157

Evening Snack

Breyers Fat-Free, Double Churned Ice Cream Sundae, with
    Walnuts, Raspberries, and Dark Chocolate (1 Serving)—p. 156

Nutritional Information Day Total

Amount Per Serving		
Calories		1544.73
Calories From Fat (28%)		435.31
		% Daily Value
Total Fat 50.09g		**77%**
Saturated Fat 14.04g		**70%**
Cholesterol 70.47mg		**23%**
Sodium 2242.62mg		**93%**
Potassium 3336.44mg		**95%**
Carbohydrates 210.07g		**70%**
Dietary Fiber 61.69g		**247%**
Sugar 73.29g		
Sugar Alcohols 0.00g		
Net Carbohydrates 148.38g		
Protein 79.32g		**159%**

For a nutritional chart for each
meal, see Appendix A, p. 231.

DAY 6

Breakfast

Multigrain Cheerios with Fruit and Nuts (1 Serving)—p. 176
Nonfat Milk (1/2 Cup)

Lunch

London Broil and Vegetable Wrap (1 Serving)—p. 172

Dinner

White Wine (1 Glass (3.5 Fl Oz))
Caesar Salad (1 Serving)—p. 158
Sesame Tuna Steaks (1 Serving)—p. 188
Apples and Brown Rice (1 Serving)—p. 152
Sautéed Kale with Garlic and Mushrooms (1 Serving)—p. 184

Evening Snack

Blackberries with Yogurt, Cinnamon, and Nutmeg Topping
(1 Serving)—p. 155

DAY 7

Nutritional Information Day Total

Amount Per Serving	
Calories	1542.14
Calories From Fat (32%)	495.11
	% Daily Value
Total Fat 57.03g	88%
Saturated Fat 10.46g	52%
Cholesterol 99.44mg	33%
Sodium 2024.56mg	84%
Potassium 3171.86mg	91%
Carbohydrates 172.37g	57%
Dietary Fiber 29.85g	119%
Sugar 57.39g	
Sugar Alcohols 0.00g	
Net Carbohydrates 142.52g	
Protein 82.61g	165%

For a nutritional chart for each
meal, see Appendix A, p. 232.

Breakfast

V–8 Calcium Enriched Vegetable Juice (8 Oz) (1 Serving)
Egg White Omelet (1 Serving)—p. 163

Lunch

Caesar Tuna Salad (1 Serving)—p. 159
Whole Wheat Pita Bread (1 Ea)
Blueberries (1/4 Cup)

Dinner

Bob's Sliced Tomatoes and Onion (1 Serving)—p. 155
Very Veggie Chili (1 Serving)—p. 199
Long-Grain Brown Rice (1 Cup)

Evening Snack

Breyers Fat-Free, Double Churned Ice Cream Sundae, with
Walnuts, Raspberries, and Dark Chocolate (1 Serving)—
p. 156

Nutritional Information Day Total

Amount Per Serving		
Calories		1398.50
Calories From Fat (32%)		443.91
		% Daily Value
Total Fat 50.99g		**78%**
Saturated Fat 8.73g		**44%**
Cholesterol 20.34mg		**7%**
Sodium 1987.68mg		**83%**
Potassium 3450.38mg		**99%**
Carbohydrates 179.76g		**60%**
Dietary Fiber 34.17g		**137%**
Sugar 51.96g		
Sugar Alcohols 0.00g		
Net Carbohydrates 145.59g		
Protein 67.73g		**135%**

For a nutritional chart for each
meal, see Appendix A, p. 233.

Breakfast

Grapefruit (1/2 Cup)
Harriet's Homemade Granola (1 Serving)—p. 170
Nonfat Milk (1/2 Cup)

Lunch

Grilled Island Shrimp Wrap (1 Serving)—p. 169
Melanie's Mango and Avocado Salad with Pomegranate
Vinaigrette Dressing (1 Serving)—p. 175

Dinner

Tossed Salad with Balsamic Vinaigrette Dressing (1 Serving)—
p. 196
Mashed Sweet Potatoes and Spinach (1 Serving)—p. 175
Spicy Garlic and Ginger Chicken (1 Serving)—p. 192
Green Snap Beans (1/2 Cup)

Evening Snack

Sliced Peaches with Raspberry, Pomegranate, and Ginger
Topping (1 Serving)—p. 189

Nutritional Information Day Total

Amount Per Serving		
Calories		1616.86
Calories From Fat (29%)		462.90
		% Daily Value
Total Fat 53.82g		**83%**
Saturated Fat 6.74g		**34%**
Cholesterol 218.89mg		**73%**
Sodium 1345.09mg		**56%**
Potassium 4449.92mg		**127%**
Carbohydrates 235.40g		**78%**
Dietary Fiber 28.43g		**114%**
Sugar 88.79g		
Sugar Alcohols 0.00g		
Net Carbohydrates 206.97g		
Protein 70.20g		**140%**

For a nutritional chart for each
meal, see Appendix A, p. 234.

Breakfast

Mixed Berries with Yogurt and Almonds (1 Serving)—p. 176

Oat Bran Bagels (1 Ea)

Lox-Smoked Salmon or Nova (1 Serving)—p. 173

Fat Free Cream Cheese (1 Oz)

Lunch

Chicken Caesar Salad (1 Serving)—p. 160

Whole Wheat Pita Bread (1 Ea)

Dinner

Sweet Potato and Leek Soup (1 Serving)—p. 193

Sol's Salmon with Horseradish and Ginger Panko Crust
    (1 Serving)—p. 190

Asparagus (10 Ea)

Peas (1/2 Cup)

Long-Grain Brown Rice (1 Cup)

Evening Snack

Breyers Fat-Free, Double Churned Ice Cream Sundae, with
    Walnuts, Raspberries, and Dark Chocolate (1 Serving)—p. 156

Nutritional Information Day Total

Amount Per Serving		
Calories		1442.17
Calories From Fat (27%)		390.93
		% Daily Value
Total Fat 45.08g		**69%**
Saturated Fat 9.49g		**47%**
Cholesterol 93.84mg		**31%**
Sodium 2808.18mg		**117%**
Potassium 2549.08mg		**73%**
Carbohydrates 187.64g		**63%**
Dietary Fiber 57.44g		**230%**
Sugar 37.70g		
Sugar Alcohols 0.00g		
Net Carbohydrates 130.20g		
Protein 80.79g		**162%**

For a nutritional chart for each
meal, see Appendix A, p. 235.

DAY 10

Breakfast

1% Milk (1/2 Cup)

Mary's Old-Fashioned Muesli with Dried Fruit (1 Serving)—
   p. 174

Margaux's Mango and Banana Smoothie (1 Serving)—p. 174

Lunch

Tropical Fruit Salad (1 Serving)—p. 196

Nonfat Plain Yogurt (1 Cup)

Ground Cinnamon (1/4 Tsp)

Dinner

Seared Tuna with Mango Salsa (1 Serving)—p. 187

Spinach and Garlic (1 Serving)—p. 193

Apples and Brown Rice (1 Serving)—p. 152

Evening Snack

Blackberries with Yogurt, Cinnamon, and Nutmeg Topping
   (1 Serving)—p. 155

Nutritional Information Day Total

Amount Per Serving		
Calories	1509.49	
Calories From Fat (29%)	437.84	
		% Daily Value
Total Fat 51.16g		79%
Saturated Fat 8.31g		42%
Cholesterol 63.36mg		21%
Sodium 1212.31mg		51%
Potassium 3296.22mg		94%
Carbohydrates 222.50g		74%
Dietary Fiber 31.42g		126%
Sugar 96.19g		
Sugar Alcohols 0.00g		
Net Carbohydrates 191.09g		
Protein 60.44g		121%

For a nutritional chart for each
meal, see Appendix A, p. 236.

Breakfast

Black Cherry Juice (1 Cup)
Omega Oatmeal (1 Serving)—p. 177
Mixed Berries with Yogurt and Almonds (1 Serving)—p. 176

Lunch

Chopped Salad with Balsamic Vinaigrette Dressing
    (1 Serving)—p. 161
Cashews, Dry Roasted Without Salt (1 Oz)

Dinner

Tossed Salad with Special Balsamic Vinaigrette Dressing
    (1 Serving)—p. 196
Ginger Chicken (1 Serving)—p. 166
Roasted Asparagus (1 Serving)—p. 181
Raisins and Brown Rice (1 Serving)—p. 180

DAY 12

Nutritional Information Day Total

Amount Per Serving		
Calories	1496.59	
Calories From Fat (31%)	467.30	
		% Daily Value
Total Fat 54.66g		**84%**
Saturated Fat 8.23g		**41%**
Cholesterol 75.91mg		**25%**
Sodium 928.12mg		**39%**
Potassium 3023.62mg		**86%**
Carbohydrates 203.93g		**68%**
Dietary Fiber 32.43g		**130%**
Sugar 62.01g		
Sugar Alcohols 0.00g		
Net Carbohydrates 171.50g		
Protein 66.05g		**132%**

For a nutritional chart for each
meal, see Appendix A, p. 237.

Breakfast

Caroline's Power Carrot Juice (1 Serving)—p. 159
Wheat Bran Muffins (1 Oz)
Veggie Frittata (1 Serving)—p. 198

Lunch

Elizabeth's Sesame Chicken Wrap (1 Serving)—p. 164
Tropical Fruit Salad (1 Serving)—p. 196

Dinner

V–8 Calcium Enriched Vegetable Juice (8 Oz) (1 Serving)
Cabbage Ginger Salad (1 Serving)—p. 158
Sirloin Steak, Fat Trimmed (2 X 3 Oz)
Beets (1/2 Cup)
Brown Rice with Turmeric (1 Serving)—p. 157

Evening Snack

Stonyfield Farm Vanilla Nonfat Frozen Yogurt (1 X 1/2 Cup)—
p. 193

Nutritional Information Day Total

Amount Per Serving	
Calories	1595.31
Calories From Fat (29%)	456.57
	% Daily Value
Total Fat 52.27g	**80%**
Saturated Fat 9.12g	**46%**
Cholesterol 223.56mg	**75%**
Sodium 1438.36mg	**60%**
Potassium 4463.84mg	**128%**
Carbohydrates 201.80g	**67%**
Dietary Fiber 24.11g	**96%**
Sugar 91.09g	
Sugar Alcohols 0.00g	
Net Carbohydrates 177.68g	
Protein 94.07g	**188%**

For a nutritional chart for each
meal, see Appendix A, p. 238.

Breakfast

Orange and Pomegranate Juice (1 Serving)—p. 178
Scrambled Egg Whites Italiano (1 Serving)—p. 184
Oat Bran Bagels (1 Ea)
Cream Cheese-Fat Free (1 Oz)

Lunch

Ginger Tuna Salad (1 Serving)—p. 168
Carrots (1/2 Cup)
Celery (1/2 Cup)
Almonds (10 Ea)

Dinner

White Wine (1 Glass (3.5 Fl Oz))
Crab Cakes (1 Serving)—p. 162
Apples and Brown Rice (1 Serving)—p. 152
Broccoli Florets (1 Cup)
Honeydew, Fresh (1 Wedge)

DAY 14

Nutritional Information Day Total

Amount Per Serving		
Calories		1683.19
Calories From Fat (23%)		384.56
		% Daily Value
Total Fat 44.27g		68%
Saturated Fat 5.53g		28%
Cholesterol 150.15mg		50%
Sodium 1836.86mg		77%
Potassium 3449.91mg		99%
Carbohydrates 211.13g		70%
Dietary Fiber 25.17g		101%
Sugar 88.94g		
Sugar Alcohols 0.00g		
Net Carbohydrates 185.95g		
Protein 100.32g		201%

For a nutritional chart for each
meal, see Appendix A, p. 239.

Breakfast

V–8 Calcium Enriched Vegetable Juice (8 Oz) (1 Serving)
Scrambled Eggs with Onions, Green Peppers (1 Serving)—p. 185
Nonfat Plain Yogurt (1/2 Cup)
Strawberries (1/4 Cup)

Lunch

Chicken Caesar Salad (1 Serving)—p. 160
Brandon's Black Bean Salsa (1 Serving)—p. 156
Whole Wheat Pita Bread (1 Ea)

Dinner

Spanish Garlic Soup (1 Serving)—p. 190
London Broil with Garlic Marinade (1 Serving)—p. 172
Roasted Asparagus (1 Serving)—p. 181
Feta and Kalamata Puree (1 Serving)—p. 164

Evening Snack

Apples and Blackberries (1/2 Cup Ea)

Nutritional Information Day Total

Amount Per Serving	
Calories	1414.07
Calories From Fat (33%)	465.28
	% Daily Value
Total Fat 52.73g	**81%**
Saturated Fat 10.92g	**55%**
Cholesterol 80.20mg	**27%**
Sodium 2551.45mg	**106%**
Potassium 4433.23mg	**127%**
Carbohydrates 135.71g	**45%**
Dietary Fiber 32.51g	**130%**
Sugar 28.72g	
Sugar Alcohols 0.00g	
Net Carbohydrates 103.20g	
Protein 101.05g	**202%**

For a nutritional chart for each
meal, see Appendix A, p. 240.

Breakfast

1% Milk (6 Fl Oz)

Multigrain Cheerios with Fruit and Nuts (1 Serving)—p. 176

Lunch

London Broil and Vegetable Wrap (1 Serving)—p. 172

Navel Orange (1 Ea)

Dinner

Salmon with Ginger-Orange Sauce (1 Serving)—p. 182

Long-Grain Brown Rice (1/2 Cup)

Sautéed Broccoli Rabe (1 Serving)—p. 183

Sesame Snow Peas with Basil (1 Serving)—p. 188

Evening Snack

Stonyfield Farm Vanilla Nonfat Frozen Yogurt (1 Serving)—
p. 193

Nutritional Information Day Total

Amount Per Serving		
Calories	1536.46	
Calories From Fat (30%)	466.73	
		% Daily Value
Total Fat 53.37g		82%
Saturated Fat 11.33g		57%
Cholesterol 120.02mg		40%
Sodium 1524.08mg		64%
Potassium 3087.90mg		88%
Carbohydrates 191.20g		64%
Dietary Fiber 29.64g		119%
Sugar 76.33g		
Sugar Alcohols 0.00g		
Net Carbohydrates 161.56g		
Protein 86.55g		173%

For a nutritional chart for each
meal, see Appendix A, p. 241.

Breakfast

V–8 Calcium Enriched Vegetable Juice (8 Oz) (1 Serving)
Omega Oatmeal (1 Serving)—p. 177
Blueberries (1/4 Cup)

Lunch

Salmon with Ginger-Orange Sauce (1 Serving)—p. 182
Cucumber Dill Salad (1 Serving)

Dinner

Sweet Potato and Leek Soup (1 Serving)—p. 193
Tossed Salad with Special Balsamic Vinaigrette Dressing
    (1 Serving)—p. 196
Portabella Mushrooms Stuffed with Crab (1 Serving)—p. 179
Peas (1/2 Cup)
Cantaloupe, Fresh (1 Cup)

Evening Snack

Ricotta and Blueberry Parfait (1 Serving)—p. 181

Nutritional Information Day Total

Amount Per Serving		
Calories		1500.54
Calories From Fat (32%)		472.71
		% Daily Value
Total Fat 54.83g		**84%**
Saturated Fat 14.97g		**75%**
Cholesterol 220.73mg		**74%**
Sodium 2004.38mg		**84%**
Potassium 5707.36mg		**163%**
Carbohydrates 179.97g		**60%**
Dietary Fiber 62.69g		**251%**
Sugar 49.99g		
Sugar Alcohols 0.00g		
Net Carbohydrates 117.29g		
Protein 90.63g		**181%**

For a nutritional chart for each
meal, see Appendix A, p. 242.

Breakfast

Black Cherry Juice (1 Cup)
Egg White Omelet (1 Serving)—p. 163
Toasted Wheat English Muffins (1 Ea)
Cream Cheese-Fat Free (1 Oz)

Lunch

V–8 Calcium Enriched Vegetable Juice (8 Oz) (1 Serving)
Ginger Tuna Salad Served on Romaine Lettuce (1 Serving)—
    p. 168
Broccoli and Garlic (1 Serving)—p. 157

Dinner

T-Bone Steak (3 Oz Serving)
Spiced Twice Baked Sweet Potato (1 Serving)—p. 191
Peas and Onions with Cumin (1 Serving)

Evening Snack

Sliced Peaches with Raspberry, Pomegranate, and Ginger
    Topping (1 Serving)—p. 189

Nutritional Information Day Total

Amount Per Serving		
Calories		1597.22
Calories From Fat (31%)		488.88
		% Daily Value
Total Fat 56.08g		**86%**
Saturated Fat 13.37g		**67%**
Cholesterol 104.39mg		**35%**
Sodium 1639.02mg		**68%**
Potassium 4023.10mg		**115%**
Carbohydrates 197.18g		**66%**
Dietary Fiber 26.86g		**107%**
Sugar 83.77g		
Sugar Alcohols 0.00g		
Net Carbohydrates 170.31g		
Protein 87.00g		**174%**

For a nutritional chart for each
meal, see Appendix A, p. 243.

Breakfast

1% Milk (1/2 Cup)
Harriet's Homemade Granola (1 Serving)—p. 170
Melons, Cantaloupe, Fresh (1 Ea)

Lunch

Chopped Salad with Special Balsamic Vinaigrette Dressing
    (1 Serving)—p. 161
Camembert (1 Oz)
Whole Wheat Crackers (5 Ea)

Dinner

Waldorf Salad (1 Serving)
Shrimp and Garlic in Lime Juice (1 Serving)—p. 189
Brandon's Black Bean Salsa (1 Serving)—p. 156
Long-Grain Brown Rice (1/2 Cup)

Evening Snack

Breyers Low Fat, Double Churned Ice Cream Sundae, with
    Walnuts, Raspberries, and Dark Chocolate (1 Serving)—p. 156

Nutritional Information Day Total

Amount Per Serving	
Calories	1751.91
Calories From Fat (27%)	480.88
	% Daily Value
Total Fat 55.85g	**86%**
Saturated Fat 14.33g	**72%**
Cholesterol 289.38mg	**96%**
Sodium 1242.28mg	**52%**
Potassium 4272.60mg	**122%**
Carbohydrates 252.18g	**84%**
Dietary Fiber 45.49g	**182%**
Sugar 109.79g	
Sugar Alcohols 0.00g	
Net Carbohydrates 206.69g	
Protein 84.91g	**170%**

For a nutritional chart for each
meal, see Appendix A, p. 244.

Breakfast

Black Cherry Juice (1 Cup)
Veggie Frittata (1 Serving)—p. 198
Toasted Whole Wheat English Muffins (1 Ea)

Lunch

Ginger Tuna Salad (1 Serving)—p. 168
Tropical Fruit Salad (1/2 Serving)—p. 196

Dinner

Caesar Salad (1 Serving)—p. 158
Tarragon Lamb Chops (1 Serving)—p. 195
Artichoke Hearts and Rice (1 Serving)—p. 152
Broccoli and Garlic (1 Serving)—p. 157

DAY 20

Nutritional Information Day Total

Amount Per Serving	
Calories	1574.27
Calories From Fat (35%)	548.33
	% Daily Value
Total Fat 63.88g	98%
Saturated Fat 9.16g	46%
Cholesterol 106.85mg	36%
Sodium 830.45mg	35%
Potassium 3134.50mg	90%
Carbohydrates 191.82g	64%
Dietary Fiber 27.47g	110%
Sugar 72.54g	
Sugar Alcohols 0.00g	
Net Carbohydrates 164.35g	
Protein 76.51g	153%

For a nutritional chart for each meal, see Appendix A, p. 245.

Breakfast

V–8 Calcium Enriched Vegetable Juice (8 Oz) (1 Serving)
Scrambled Eggs with Onions, Green Peppers (1 Serving)—p. 185
Toasted Whole Wheat Bread (1 Slice)
Unsalted Butter (1 Pat)

Lunch

Bob's Sliced Tomato and Onion (1 Serving)—p. 155
Seafood Salad (1 Serving)—p. 185
Cantaloupe, Fresh (1 Cup)

Dinner

White Wine (1 Glass (3.5 Fl Oz))
Sweet Potato and Leek Soup (1 Serving)—p. 193
Panko Chicken with Black Cherry Sauce (1 Serving)—p. 178
Brown Rice with Turmeric (1 Serving)—p. 157
Feta and Kalamata Puree (1 Serving)—p. 164

Evening Snack

Chocolate Covered Strawberries (1 Serving)—p. 161

DAY 21

Nutritional Information Day Total

Amount Per Serving	
Calories	1530.49
Calories From Fat (31%)	479.06
	% Daily Value
Total Fat 54.11g	83%
Saturated Fat 13.01g	65%
Cholesterol 175.98mg	59%
Sodium 2030.47mg	85%
Potassium 4473.43mg	128%
Carbohydrates 164.77g	55%
Dietary Fiber 54.84g	219%
Sugar 64.91g	
Sugar Alcohols 0.00g	
Net Carbohydrates 109.94g	
Protein 84.42g	169%

For a nutritional chart for each
meal, see Appendix A, p. 246.

Breakfast

V-8 Calcium Enriched Vegetable Juice (8 Oz) (1 Serving)
Egg White Omelet (1 Serving)—p. 163
Cantaloupe, Fresh (1 Serving)

Lunch

Gazpacho (1 Serving)—p. 166
Hummus (1 Serving)—p. 171
Celery (Cup)
Carrots (1 Cup)
Whole Wheat Pita Bread (1 Ea)

Dinner

Tossed Salad with Special Balsamic Vinaigrette Dressing
  (1 Serving)—p. 196
Seafood Stew (1 Serving)—p. 186
Long-Grain Brown Rice (1 Cup)

DAY 22

Nutritional Information Day Total

Amount Per Serving		
Calories		1542.22
Calories From Fat (32%)		496.07
		% Daily Value
Total Fat 56.95g		**88%**
Saturated Fat 6.01g		**30%**
Cholesterol 114.71mg		**38%**
Sodium 2679.41mg		**112%**
Potassium 4436.99mg		**127%**
Carbohydrates 191.69g		**64%**
Dietary Fiber 30.92g		**124%**
Sugar 53.13g		
Sugar Alcohols 0.00g		
Net Carbohydrates 160.77g		
Protein 77.24g		**154%**

For a nutritional chart for each
meal, see Appendix A, p. 247.

Breakfast

Nonfat Milk (1/2 Cup)
Multigrain Cheerios with Fruit and Nuts (1 Serving)—p. 176

Lunch

Melanie's Mango and Avocado Salad with Pomegranate
   Vinaigrette Dressing (1 Serving)—p. 175
Seafood Salad (1 Serving)—p. 185

Dinner

Salad with Ginger Dressing (1 Serving)—p. 167
London Broil with Garlic Marinade (1 Serving)—p. 172
Horseradish Sauce (1 Serving)—p. 171
Cauliflower (1 X 1/2 Cup, (1" Pieces))
Mashed Sweet Potatoes and Spinach (1 Serving)—p. 175

DAY 23

Nutritional Information Day Total

Amount Per Serving		
Calories	1488.02	
Calories From Fat (34%)	499.77	
		% Daily Value
Total Fat 58.19g		**90%**
Saturated Fat 10.27g		**51%**
Cholesterol 142.00mg		**47%**
Sodium 1394.97mg		**58%**
Potassium 5071.12mg		**145%**
Carbohydrates 189.12g		**63%**
Dietary Fiber 24.13g		**97%**
Sugar 55.65g		
Sugar Alcohols 0.00g		
Net Carbohydrates 164.99g		
Protein 73.22g		**146%**

For a nutritional chart for each
meal, see Appendix A, p. 248.

Breakfast

Cinnamon Yogurt (1 Serving)—p. 162
Omega Oatmeal (1 Serving)—p. 177

Lunch

V–8 Calcium Enriched Vegetable Juice (8 Oz) (1 Serving)
London Broil and Vegetable Wrap (1 Serving)—p. 172
Cantaloupe, Fresh (1 Cup)

Dinner

Chopped Salad with Special Balsamic Vinaigrette Dressing
    (1 Serving)—p. 161
Grapefruit (1/2 Fruit (3–3/4" Dia))
Mustard Salmon (1 Serving)—p. 177
Long-Grain Brown Rice (1/2 Cup)
Roasted Asparagus (1 Serving)—p. 181

DAY 24

Nutritional Information Day Total

Amount Per Serving		
Calories	1524.35	
Calories From Fat (26%)	400.87	
		% Daily Value
Total Fat 45.90g		**71%**
Saturated Fat 12.20g		**61%**
Cholesterol 117.71mg		**39%**
Sodium 1755.44mg		**73%**
Potassium 4520.09mg		**129%**
Carbohydrates 201.25g		**67%**
Dietary Fiber 33.82g		**135%**
Sugar 43.22g		
Sugar Alcohols 0.00g		
Net Carbohydrates 167.43g		
Protein 91.50g		**183%**

For a nutritional chart for each
meal, see Appendix A, p. 249.

Breakfast

V–8 Calcium Enriched Vegetable Juice (8 Oz) (1 Serving)
Scrambled Eggs with Onions, Green Peppers (1 Serving)—p. 185
Toasted Whole Wheat Bread (1 Slice)
Unsalted Butter (1 Pat)

Lunch

Sweet Potato and Leek Soup (1 Serving)—p. 193
Caesar Tuna Salad (1 Serving)—p. 159
Whole Wheat Pita Bread (1 Ea)

Dinner

Tossed Salad with Special Balsamic Vinaigrette Dressing
(1 Serving)—p. 196
Very Veggie Chili (1 Serving)—p. 199
Long-Grain Brown Rice (1/2 Cup)
Healthy Baked Garlic Tortilla Chips (1 Serving)—p. 170

Evening Snack

Breyers Fat-Free, Double Churned Ice Cream Sundae, with
Walnuts, Raspberries, and Dark Chocolate (1 Serving)—p. 156

Nutritional Information Day Total

Amount Per Serving	
Calories	1552.35
Calories From Fat (33%)	519.57
	% Daily Value
Total Fat 59.49g	**92%**
Saturated Fat 12.59g	**63%**
Cholesterol 32.35mg	**11%**
Sodium 2661.03mg	**111%**
Potassium 3677.28mg	**105%**
Carbohydrates 191.45g	**64%**
Dietary Fiber 60.96g	**244%**
Sugar 44.71g	
Sugar Alcohols 0.00g	
Net Carbohydrates 130.49g	
Protein 74.14g	**148%**

For a nutritional chart for each
meal, see Appendix A, p. 250.

Breakfast

V–8 Calcium Enriched Vegetable Juice (8 Oz) (1 Serving)
Mary's Old-Fashioned Muesli with Dried Fruit (1 Serving)—
p. 174
Nonfat Milk (1/2 Cup)

Lunch

Tropical Fruit Salad (1 Serving)—p. 196
Avocado Pita Sandwich (1 Serving)—p. 153

Dinner

Tossed Salad with Special Balsamic Vinaigrette Dressing
(1 Serving)—p. 196
Garlic Shrimp in White Wine over Whole Wheat Linguini
(1 Serving)—p. 165

Evening Snack

Sliced Peaches with Raspberry, Pomegranate and Ginger
Topping (1 Serving)—p. 189

Nutritional Information Day Total

Amount Per Serving		
Calories		1587.40
Calories From Fat (37%)		594.51
		% Daily Value
Total Fat 69.74g		**107%**
Saturated Fat 7.69g		**38%**
Cholesterol 209.64mg		**70%**
Sodium 1328.36mg		**55%**
Potassium 3953.03mg		**113%**
Carbohydrates 202.16g		**67%**
Dietary Fiber 36.07g		**144%**
Sugar 85.73g		
Sugar Alcohols 0.00g		
Net Carbohydrates 166.10g		
Protein 55.05g		**110%**

For a nutritional chart for each
meal, see Appendix A, p. 251.

Breakfast

Margaux's Mango and Banana Smoothie (1 Serving)—p. 174
Scrambled Eggs with Onions, Green Peppers (1 Serving)—p. 185

Lunch

Cabbage Ginger Salad (1 Serving)—p. 158
Grilled Island Shrimp Wrap (1 Serving)—p. 169

Dinner

V–8 Calcium Enriched Vegetable Juice (8 Oz) (1 Serving)
Caesar Salad (1 Serving)—p. 158
Panko Chicken with Black Cherry Sauce (1 Serving)—p. 178
Sesame Snow Peas with Basil (1 Serving)—p. 188
Yellow Squash with Lemon (1 Serving)—p. 200

DAY 27

Nutritional Information Day Total

Amount Per Serving	
Calories	1455.61
Calories From Fat (40%)	585.71
	% Daily Value
Total Fat 67.53g	**104%**
Saturated Fat 7.98g	**40%**
Cholesterol 246.81mg	**82%**
Sodium 1685.03mg	**70%**
Potassium 3939.58mg	**113%**
Carbohydrates 133.16g	**44%**
Dietary Fiber 27.51g	**110%**
Sugar 57.82g	
Sugar Alcohols 0.00g	
Net Carbohydrates 105.66g	
Protein 92.30g	**185%**

For a nutritional chart for each
meal, see Appendix A, p. 252.

Breakfast

Orange and Pomegranate Juice (1 Serving)—p. 178
Omega Oatmeal (1 Serving)—p. 177

Lunch

Greek Salad (1 Serving)—p. 168
Pita Bread (1 Ea)

Dinner

White Wine (1 Glass (3.5 Fl Oz))
Salmon with Ginger-Orange Sauce (1 Serving)—p. 182
Baby Portabella Mushrooms (Crimini) with Artichoke Hearts
 (1 Serving)—p. 153
Sweet Potato Hash (1 Serving)—p. 194
Chocolate Covered Strawberries (1 Serving)—p. 161

DAY 28

Nutritional Information Day Total

Amount Per Serving	
Calories	1596.73
Calories From Fat (37%)	584.44
	% Daily Value
Total Fat 66.11g	**102%**
Saturated Fat 14.13g	**71%**
Cholesterol 70.00mg	**23%**
Sodium 1113.97mg	**46%**
Potassium 2624.75mg	**75%**
Carbohydrates 194.32g	**65%**
Dietary Fiber 23.59g	**94%**
Sugar 64.29g	
Sugar Alcohols 0.00g	
Net Carbohydrates 170.72g	
Protein 47.70g	**95%**

For a nutritional chart for each
meal, see Appendix A, p. 253.

CHAPTER

Great Recipes

I can personally attest to the mouthwatering deliciousness of the ninety-one recipes listed below because I have prepared and tasted every one of them in my own kitchen. I created some, but many were given to me by my wonderful patients. The recipes have also been reviewed by a registered dietitian to ensure their healthfulness. (For a complete shopping list of all the ingredients you'll need, see Appendix B.) So without further ado . . . enjoy!

Apples and Brown Rice

Serves 2

1 cup brown rice
2 cups water
1 apple, chopped
1 tbs cinnamon

- Put rice, cinnamon, and apple into a medium-sized pot.
- Add water.
- Bring to a boil and then cover with a tight fitting lid. Reduce heat and let simmer until rice has absorbed all of the liquid and is tender, about 30 minutes.

Nutrition Facts   Nutrition (per serving): 177.0 calories; 5% calories from fat; 1.2g total fat; 0.0mg cholesterol; 14.0mg sodium; 184.5mg potassium; 41.0g carbohydrates; 6.4g fiber; 12.4g sugar; 2.9g protein.

Artichoke Hearts and Rice

Serves 2

1 tbs olive oil
2 cloves garlic, minced
1/4 cup onion, chopped
1/4 cup sweet red pepper, chopped
1/4 cup artichoke hearts, drained and chopped
1 tbs fresh lemon juice
1/4 tsp paprika
1 dash red pepper flakes
1 tbs chopped walnuts
1 cup cooked brown rice, chilled

- Heat olive oil in medium frying pan.
- Cook garlic until soft, do not brown.
- Add onion, sweet red peppers, paprika, lemon juice, red pepper and artichoke hearts. Cook until onions and red peppers are soft.
- Fold mixture and walnuts into cooked brown rice.

Nutrition Facts Nutrition (per serving): 222.9 calories; 39% calories from fat; 10.2g total fat; 0.0mg cholesterol; 27.3mg sodium; 229.0mg potassium; 30.0g carbohydrates; 4.1g fiber; 2.3g sugar; 4.5g protein.

Avocado Pita Sandwich
Serves 2

1 avocado, sliced
1/2 cup tomatoes, chopped
1 cucumber, coarsely chopped
1/2 cup button mushrooms, sliced
2 whole wheat pita bread pockets
1 tbs Special Balsamic Vinaigrette Dressing

- Dice ripe avocado, tomatoes, cucumber, and mushrooms.
- Fold above ingredients, add dressing, and fill warm pita bread.

Nutrition Facts Nutrition (per serving): 266.5 calories; 54% calories from fat; 17.3g total fat; 0.0mg cholesterol; 160.5mg sodium; 744.2mg potassium; 27.0g carbohydrates; 9.1g fiber; 2.9g sugar; 5.8g protein.

Baby Portabella Mushrooms (Crimini) with Artichoke Hearts
Serves 3

2 tbs olive oil
6 cloves garlic, sliced
3 cups baby portabella mushrooms (crimini), sliced
1 can artichoke hearts (drained)
1 tbs fresh basil
1 tbs fresh oregano
5 oz fresh spinach
1 tbs flaxseed meal
1 tbs lemon juice
salt to taste

- Heat olive oil in large skillet.
- Sauté garlic for about 2 minutes, do not brown.
- Add basil, oregano, salt, mushrooms, and artichoke hearts, sauté until mushrooms are soft.
- Add spinach and cook until wilted.
- Add lemon juice and flaxseed meal.

Nutrition Facts   Nutrition (per serving): 169.9 calories; 52% calories from fat; 10.2g total fat; 0.0mg cholesterol; 166.5mg sodium; 897.1mg potassium; 16.5g carbohydrates; 6.8g fiber; 1.6g sugar; 6.8g protein.

Baked Chicken with Garlic

Serves 2

2 chicken breast (free-range) halves (boneless, skin removed)
1 tsp garlic powder
1 tsp fresh oregano (finely chopped)
1 tsp fresh basil (finely chopped)

- Combine garlic powder, oregano, and basil.
- Pat onto chicken breast halves.
- Preheat oven to 450 degrees.
- Bake chicken for 40 minutes, or until done.

Nutrition Facts   Nutrition (per serving): 138.5 calories; 10% calories from fat; 1.6g total fat; 68.4mg cholesterol; 77.4mg sodium; 352.9mg potassium; 1.9g carbohydrates; 0.7g fiber; 0.4g sugar; 27.7g protein.

Black Cherry Sauce

Serves 8

1/4 cup cherries (frozen are fine)
3/4 cup black cherry juice
1 tbs fresh lemon juice
1 tsp arrowroot
1 tbs orange juice
1 tsp Dijon mustard
1 dash cayenne pepper

- Defrost frozen cherries and pulse in blender until slightly broken.
- Remove 2 tablespoons of black cherry juice and put aside. Slowly heat remainder of juice over low heat.
- Add cherries, lemon juice, orange juice, mustard, and cayenne pepper to warm cherry juice.
- Mix reserved cherry juice with arrowroot. Slowly add to warm cherry juice mixture, stirring continuously until thickened.
- Remove from heat. Can be used warm.
- Store remainder in refrigerator in covered plastic container.

Nutrition Facts   Nutrition (per serving): 22.2 calories; 2% calories from fat; 0.1g total fat; 0.0mg cholesterol; 11.7mg sodium; 38.9mg potassium; 5.4g carbohydrates; 0.1g fiber; 3.6g sugar; 0.3g protein.

Blackberries with Yogurt, Cinnamon and Nutmeg Topping

Serves 1

1/2 cup blackberries
1 tbs Yogurt Cinnamon and Nutmeg Topping (see recipe)

- Combine blackberries with Yogurt Cinnamon and Nutmeg Topping.

Nutrition Facts   Nutrition (per serving): 49.6 calories; 10% calories from fat; 0.6g total fat; 1.0mg cholesterol; 14.3mg sodium; 163.4mg potassium; 10.1g carbohydrates; 4.0g fiber; 6.4g sugar; 2.0g protein.

Bob's Sliced Tomato and Onion

Serves 1

1 medium tomato, sliced
1 small onion, thinly sliced
2 tbs Special Balsamic Vinaigrette Dressing
1 tbs fresh basil, chopped

- Arrange tomato, alternating with onion.
- Drizzle dressing over tomato and onion.
- Sprinkle chopped basil over tomato and onion.

Nutrition Facts   Nutrition (per serving): 182.1 calories; 59% calories from fat; 12.4g total fat; 0.0mg cholesterol; 11.7mg sodium; 503.5mg potassium; 17.7g carbohydrates; 3.7g fiber; 8.4g sugar; 2.6g protein.

Brandon's Black Bean Salsa

Serves 4

1 tbs walnut oil
1 bunch scallions, trimmed (green and white parts)
1/2 cup yellow pepper
1/2 cup red onion
1 1/2 tsp ground cumin
2 cloves garlic, chopped
2 tbs chopped fresh cilantro
1 1/2 tbs fresh lime juice
1 can (15-ounce) black beans, drained and rinsed well
1 tbs flaxseed meal
freshly ground black pepper, and salt to taste

- Finely dice red onion, yellow peppers, and scallions to about the same size.
- Heat the oil in a medium saucepan over medium heat.
- Add scallions, yellow peppers, red onion, garlic, and cumin and cook for 3 minutes.
- Remove from heat and stir in the lime juice.
- Add the beans, cilantro, flaxseed meal, salt, and pepper and toss to coat.

Nutrition Facts   Nutrition (per serving): 204.5 calories; 20% calories from fat; 4.9g total fat; 0.0mg cholesterol; 256.4mg sodium; 531.8mg potassium; 31.7g carbohydrates; 11.0g fiber; 0.7g sugar; 10.9g protein.

Breyers Fat-Free, Double Churned Ice Cream Sundae with Walnuts, Raspberries, and Dark Chocolate

Serves 1

1/2 cup Breyers Fat-free Ice Cream – Double Churned
1 tbs walnuts, chopped

1/4 oz, shaved, 70% dark chocolate
1/4 cup raspberries

- Top ice cream with walnuts, shaved dark chocolate, and raspberries.

Nutrition Facts   Nutrition (per serving): 210.0 calories; 44% calories from fat; 10.8g total fat; 5.5mg cholesterol; 60.5mg sodium; 79.5mg potassium; 26.9g carbohydrates; 6.0g fiber; 18.3g sugar; 4.5g protein.

Broccoli and Garlic

Serves 2

2 cups broccoli
6 cloves garlic, chopped
1/2 tsp walnut oil
1/2 cup walnuts

- Steam broccoli until bright green and slightly firm.
- Drain broccoli.
- Lightly sauté garlic in walnut oil, do not brown.
- Add broccoli to sautéed garlic and mix.
- Sprinkle chopped walnuts over broccoli and garlic mixture.
- Serve immediately.

Nutrition Facts   Nutrition (per serving): 234.5 calories; 73% calories from fat; 20.5g total fat; 0.0mg cholesterol; 21.3mg sodium; 395.8mg potassium; 10.7g carbohydrates; 2.1g fiber; 0.9g sugar; 7.1g protein.

Brown Rice with Turmeric

Serves 2

1 cup brown rice, cooked
1/4 tsp turmeric
1/4 cup onion
1 clove garlic, chopped
1 tbs flaxseed meal

- To one cup of cooked brown rice add turmeric and mix well.

- Spray pan with nonstick vegetable spray. Sauté onion and garlic.
- Add onion and garlic to brown rice mixture.
- Add flaxseed meal to brown rice. Mix well.

Nutrition Facts   Nutrition (per serving): 136.5 calories; 12% calories from fat; 2.1g total fat; 0.0mg cholesterol; 6.3mg sodium; 98.6mg potassium; 26.3g carbohydrates; 3.3g fiber; 1.2g sugar; 3.6g protein.

Cabbage Ginger Salad
Serves 2

1 cup red cabbage, chopped
1 large scallion, chopped
1 medium tomato, seeded and sliced
2 tbs Ginger Dressing (see recipe)

- Combine cabbage, scallions, and tomato in a bowl.
- Toss with ginger dressing.

Nutrition Facts   Nutrition (per serving): 62.1 calories; 44% calories from fat; 3.6g total fat; 0.0mg cholesterol; 265.0mg sodium; 300.3mg potassium; 8.3g carbohydrates; 2.3g fiber; 3.4g sugar; 1.9g protein.

Caesar Salad
Serves 4

1 head romaine lettuce, shredded
1/4 cup walnuts, finely chopped
1 anchovy from can, finely chopped
4 cloves garlic, chopped
dressing
2 tbs flaxseed oil
2 tbs balsamic vinegar

- Combine lettuce, walnuts, anchovy, and garlic into bowl.
- Whisk flaxseed oil and vinegar.
- Toss salad with dressing.

Nutrition Facts   Nutrition (per serving): 144.4 calories; 72% calories from fat; 12.2g total fat; 1.7mg cholesterol; 86.7mg sodium; 450.0mg potassium; 7.6g carbohydrates; 3.8g fiber; 2.1g sugar; 3.8g protein.

Caesar Tuna Salad

Serves 2

1 can tuna, light or white, with oil drained
2 servings Caesar Salad (see recipe)

- Top Caesar Salad with one can of drained tuna.

Nutrition Facts   Nutrition (per serving): 288.9 calories; 55% calories from fat; 18.2g total fat; 14.8mg cholesterol; 345.1mg sodium; 601.1mg potassium; 7.6g carbohydrates; 3.8g fiber; 2.1g sugar; 25.1g protein.

Caroline's Power Carrot Juice

Serves 1

1 cup carrot juice, fresh
1 tbs flaxseed oil

- Mix flaxseed oil with fresh carrot juice.

Nutrition Facts   Nutrition (per serving): 214.6 calories; 57% calories from fat; 14.0g total fat; 0.0mg cholesterol; 68.4mg sodium; 689.1mg potassium; 21.9g carbohydrates; 1.9g fiber; 9.2g sugar; 2.2g protein.

Cauliflower—Steamed

Serves 1

1 cup cauliflower

- Steam cauliflower until tender.

Nutrition Facts   Nutrition (per serving): 25.0 calories; 3% calories from fat; 0.1g total fat; 0.0mg cholesterol; 30.0mg sodium; 303.0mg potassium; 5.3g carbohydrates; 2.5g fiber; 2.4g sugar; 2.0g protein.

Chicken Caesar Salad

Serves 4

1 head romaine lettuce
1/4 cup walnuts (chopped)
1 anchovy from can
4 cloves garlic, minced
1/2 chicken breast (free-range), baked and thinly sliced
3 tbs Special Balsamic Vinaigrette Dressing (see recipe)

- Coarsely chop romaine lettuce.
- Mash anchovy into bowl.
- Add romaine lettuce, walnuts, and minced garlic to bowl and mix with anchovy.
- Toss with Special Vinaigrette Dressing.
- Top with sliced baked chicken.

Nutrition Facts   Nutrition (per serving): 156.9 calories; 56% calories from fat; 10.3g total fat; 18.8mg cholesterol; 105.9mg sodium; 524.9mg potassium; 7.7g carbohydrates; 3.9g fiber; 2.1g sugar; 10.7g protein.

Chicken Pita Sandwich

Serves 2

1 cup baked chicken with thyme, sage, and cumin, chopped
1/4 cup tomatoes
1/2 cucumber
1/4 cup white mushrooms
2 whole wheat pita bread pockets
1 tbs Balsamic Vinaigrette Dressing
1/4 cup alfalfa sprouts

- Dice baked chicken (can use any chicken recipe from night before).
- Dice tomatoes, cucumber, and mushrooms.
- Combine chicken, tomatoes, cucumber, mushrooms, and dressing.
- Open pita bread and stuff with chicken/vegetable mixture. Top with alfalfa sprouts.

Nutrition Facts   Nutrition (per serving): 200.9 calories; 25% calories from fat; 5.9g total fat; 34.2mg cholesterol; 295.7mg sodium; 348.4mg potassium; 20.4g carbohydrates; 3.1g fiber; 1.5g sugar; 17.7g protein.

Chocolate Covered Strawberries

Serves 2

6 strawberries
1 serving dark chocolate, 70% cocoa

- Melt dark chocolate in microwave.
- Dip strawberries into melted chocolate and allow to cool.

Nutrition Facts   Nutrition (per serving): 127.3 calories; 64% calories from fat; 8.7g total fat; 1.0mg cholesterol; 10.5mg sodium; 82.6mg potassium; 10.6g carbohydrates; 2.1g fiber; 8.1g sugar; 0.4g protein.

Chopped Salad with Special Balsamic Vinaigrette Dressing

Serves 4

1 head iceberg or Boston bibb lettuce
1/2 can artichoke hearts
1 can hearts of palm
1 ripe avocado
1 cup tomatoes
1 large cucumber
4 large scallions
1/2 cup radishes
1/4 cup toasted pignolias (pine nuts)
4 tbs Special Balsamic Vinaigrette Dressing (see recipe)

- Drain artichoke hearts and hearts of palm.
- Chop lettuce, avocado, tomatoes, cucumber, scallions, radishes, artichoke hearts, and hearts of palm.
- Combine all ingredients and toss with Special Balsamic Vinaigrette Dressing.

Nutrition Facts   Nutrition (per serving): 213.8 calories; 56% calories from fat; 14.2g total fat; 0.0mg cholesterol; 122.6mg sodium; 946.9mg potassium; 20.7g carbohydrates; 10.2g fiber; 5.6g sugar; 6.3g protein.

Cinnamon Yogurt

Serves 1

1 cup yogurt nonfat, plain
1/4 tsp cinnamon, ground

- Mix cinnamon into one cup of yogurt.

Nutrition Facts   Nutrition (per serving): 156.6 calories; 21% calories from fat; 3.8g total fat; 14.9mg cholesterol; 172.1mg sodium; 575.7mg potassium; 17.7g carbohydrates; 0.3g fiber; 0.0g sugar; 12.9g protein.

Crab Cakes

Serves 1

1 can lump crabmeat
2 egg whites
1/2 tsp Dijon mustard
1 tbs parsley, chopped
1 tbs flaxseed meal
1 tsp fresh lemon juice
1/2 tsp Worcestershire sauce
1/4 cup Panko whole wheat breadcrumbs

- Combine first seven ingredients in medium bowl, gently folding in crab-meat, and mix.
- Add enough breadcrumbs to shape mixture into small cakes. Coat with additional crumbs, if desired.
- Place on a baking sheet (sprayed with nonstick cooking oil) and bake in 400 degree oven for twenty minutes or until golden, flipping cakes over once during cooking.

Nutrition Facts   Nutrition (per serving): 301.6 calories; 15% calories from fat; 5.5g total fat; 111.3mg cholesterol; 782.8mg sodium; 679.9mg potassium; 23.2g carbohydrates; 3.4g fiber; 2.3g sugar; 38.3g protein.

Egg White Omelet

Serves 1

4 egg whites
1/4 tsp turmeric
1/8 tsp salt
1/4 cup onions
1 tsp walnut oil
2 cloves garlic
1/8 tsp black pepper, fresh ground
1/4 cup red peppers
1 tsp parsley, chopped
2 oz. water

- Separate 4 eggs, saving the egg whites.
- Add turmeric, salt, pepper, and water into egg whites. Whisk until white peaks form.
- Heat walnut oil in nonstick frying pan.
- Add garlic and cook until fragrant.
- Sauté onions and red peppers until tender. Remove mixture from pan and set aside.
- Place pan on low heat and add egg white mixture.
- Once eggs set up, spread onions and peppers mixture over half of omelet.
- Fold omelet in half, cook for 2 more minutes.
- Slide on plate, sprinkle parsley on top.

Nutrition Facts   Nutrition (per serving): 146.1 calories; 30% calories from fat; 5.0g total fat; 0.0mg cholesterol; 526.6mg sodium; 400.5mg potassium; 9.5g carbohydrates; 1.8g fiber; 4.3g sugar; 15.7g protein.

Elizabeth's Sesame Chicken Wrap

Serves 1

1 3-oz-serving sesame chicken, diced
1/2 cup iceberg or Boston bibb lettuce, shredded
2 teaspoons cilantro, chopped
1/4 cup radishes, sliced
1 whole wheat tortilla (pre-packaged is fine)
1 serving Balsamic Vinaigrette Dressing

- Dice sesame chicken.
- Combine chicken with shredded lettuce, sliced radishes, and chopped cilantro.
- Divide mixture, spoon into middle of tortilla wrap.
- Drizzle vinaigrette dressing over chicken mixture and fold tortilla into wrap.

Nutrition Facts   Nutrition (per serving): 143.4 calories; 27% calories from fat; 4.5g total fat; 64.6mg cholesterol; 68.1mg sodium; 201.3mg potassium; 15.3g carbohydrates; 2.2g fiber; 1.3g sugar; 11.0g protein.

Feta and Kalamata Puree

Serves 4

1 lb cauliflower flowerets
1/4 cup yogurt, nonfat, plain
2 cloves garlic, minced
2 scallions, chopped
2 tbs feta cheese
1 tbs parsley, chopped
4 kalamata olives, chopped

- Microwave cauliflower until soft (about 4 minutes), or you can also steam it.
- Puree cauliflower in food processor with yogurt, garlic, scallions, and feta cheese.
- Garnish with chopped parsley and kalamata olives.

Nutrition Facts   Nutrition (per serving): 74.5 calories; 28% calories from fat; 2.4g total fat; 5.1mg cholesterol; 168.5mg sodium; 520.0mg potassium; 10.6g carbohydrates; 4.0g fiber; 4.0g sugar; 4.7g protein.

Garlic Shrimp in White Wine over Whole Wheat Linguini

Serves 4

1 lb shrimp

1 oz walnut oil

1 oz olive oil

10 cloves garlic, minced

3 cups plum tomatoes, diced

1 cup sliced baby portabella mushrooms (crimini)

1/2 cup white wine (I prefer a Chardonnay)

6 tbs fresh parsley

1 tbs fresh oregano

2 tbs fresh basil

1/4 tsp red pepper flakes

1/2 tsp salt

1 cup whole wheat linguini

- Heat olive oil and walnut oil and add minced garlic, and half the parsley.
- Cook garlic and parsley for 2 minutes, until garlic is slightly soft, but not brown.
- Add tomatoes, basil, oregano, salt, red pepper flakes, and mushrooms. Cook until tomatoes are soft, about 5 to 10 minutes.
- Add wine to deglaze, and cook about 10 minutes until alcohol is burned off.
- Add shrimp. Stir and cover shrimp until they turn pinkish-red.
- Add remainder of parsley and serve over linguini.

Nutrition Facts   Nutrition (per serving): 365.3 calories; 38% calories from fat; 15.9g total fat; 207.2mg cholesterol; 544.0mg sodium; 718.6mg potassium; 23.4g carbohydrates; 2.9g fiber; 4.3g sugar; 26.9g protein.

Gazpacho

Serves 2

2 cups tomato juice
1/2 cucumber, peeled and chopped
1 tomato, chopped
1/2 green pepper, chopped
1 tsp onion, chopped
2 tbs flaxseed oil
1/2 cup scallion, chopped
1 tsp fresh oregano, chopped
1 tbs fresh parsley, minced
2 cloves garlic, chopped
1 tbs fresh basil, chopped
2 tbs red wine vinegar
1 tbs lime juice
1 dash Tabasco

- Blend all the ingredients in a blender or food processor until smooth.
- Add salt to taste.

Nutrition Facts   Nutrition (per serving): 220.9 calories; 56% calories from fat; 14.3g total fat; 0.0mg cholesterol; 183.4mg sodium; 931.9mg potassium; 22.0g carbohydrates; 5.0g fiber; 13.8g sugar; 3.6g protein.

Ginger Chicken

Serves 4

4 pieces of free-range chicken breasts (skinless and boneless)
1 tbs walnut oil
1 tbs tamari
1 tbs fresh ginger, grated
1/2 tbs fresh lemon juice
2 cloves garlic, minced

- Combine walnut oil, tamari, ginger, lemon, and garlic in mixing bowl.
- Clean chicken, pat dry, and put in Zip-lock plastic bag.

- Add walnut oil, tamari, ginger, lemon, and garlic mixture to chicken. Remove air, close bag. Put in refrigerator for one to two hours.
- Remove chicken from plastic bag and bake at 420 degrees for 40 minutes, or until done.

Nutrition Facts   Nutrition (per serving): 166.5 calories; 26% calories from fat; 4.9g total fat; 68.4mg cholesterol; 328.5mg sodium; 325.0mg potassium; 1.2g carbohydrates; 0.1g fiber; 0.2g sugar; 27.8g protein.

Ginger Chicken Wrap
Serves 1

1 Ginger Chicken serving (see recipe)
1/2 cup tomatoes
1 cucumber
1/2 cup mushrooms
1 whole wheat pita bread pocket

- Shred chicken.
- Dice tomatoes, cucumber, and mushrooms.
- Combine chicken and vegetables.
- Fill pita with chicken and vegetable mixture.

Nutrition Facts   Nutrition (per serving): 140.4 calories; 19% calories from fat; 3.1g total fat; 34.2mg cholesterol; 243.2mg sodium; 439.1mg potassium; 12.1g carbohydrates; 2.3g fiber; 2.6g sugar; 16.6g protein.

Ginger Dressing
Serves 8

1 tsp grated fresh ginger
2 cloves garlic, chopped
1/4 tbs rice vinegar
1 tbs tamari
1/4 tbs Flaxseed Oil

- Mix ginger, garlic, and tamari into vinegar.
- Slowly pour flaxseed oil into vinegar mixture. Stir constantly until emulsion forms.

Nutrition Facts   Nutrition (per serving): 6.5 calories; 52% calories from fat; 0.4g total fat; 0.0mg cholesterol; 125.9mg sodium; 12.2mg potassium; 0.6g carbohydrates; 0.0g fiber; 0.1g sugar; 0.3g protein.

Ginger Tuna Salad Served on Romaine Lettuce

Serves 2

1 can tuna, with oil drained
2 tbs scallions
1/2 tsp fresh ginger, peeled and grated
2 water chestnuts, finely chopped
1 tsp flaxseed oil
1/4 tbs fresh parsley
1/4 tbs sesame seeds, toasted
4 leaves romaine lettuce, whole

- Drain tuna.
- Chop scallions, parsley, and water chestnuts.
- Mix tuna, scallions, parsley, water chestnuts, flaxseed oil, sesame seeds, and ginger in a bowl.
- Wash and dry lettuce.
- Spread tuna mixture down middle of each romaine lettuce leaf.

Nutrition Facts   Nutrition (per serving): 256.2 calories; 19% calories from fat; 5.6g total fat; 36.1mg cholesterol; 64.8mg sodium; 550.9mg potassium; 29.5g carbohydrates; 6.4g fiber; 6.0g sugar; 22.9g protein.

Greek Salad

Serves 6

6 plum tomatoes
2 cucumbers
1 red onion
4 tsp fresh lemon juice
8 kalamata olives
1 1/2 tbs fresh oregano, chopped
1 cup feta cheese, crumbled
1/4 cup flaxseed oil vinaigrette dressing

- Coarsely chop tomatoes.
- Peel and coarsely chop cucumbers.
- Thinly slice onion.
- Dice kalamata olives.
- Combine above ingredients, add oregano, feta cheese, and lemon juice and toss with dressing.

Nutrition Facts   Nutrition (per serving): 115.1 calories; 56% calories from fat; 7.3g total fat; 22.3mg cholesterol; 364.2mg sodium; 312.8mg potassium; 8.4g carbohydrates; 2.2g fiber; 4.1g sugar; 5.0g protein.

Grilled Island Shrimp Wrap

Serves 2

1/2 lb shrimp (cleaned, deveined, with tails removed)
1 tbs olive oil
1/2 cup green peppers, diced
1/2 cup snow peas
2 tsps fresh chopped cilantro
1 tsp curry powder
2 tortillas, whole wheat (pre-packaged)

- Heat oil in pan.
- Sauté green peppers and snow peas until tender.
- Add shrimp, curry powder, and cilantro. Cook until shrimp are pink.
- Divide shrimp into two portions and spread into center of each tortilla.
- Fold tortilla into wrap.

Nutrition Facts   Nutrition (per serving): 259.0 calories; 32% calories from fat; 9.6g total fat; 172.4mg cholesterol; 174.3mg sodium; 387.7mg potassium; 17.4g carbohydrates; 3.0g fiber; 1.9g sugar; 25.7g protein.

Harriet's Homemade Granola

Serves 4

2 cups oatmeal (steel-cut, rolled)
1/4 cup brown sugar
1/4 tsp cinnamon
1/4 cup walnuts, chopped
1/4 cup raisins
1/4 cup honey
4 tbs flaxseed meal

- Preheat oven to 325 degrees.
- In a bowl, combine oats, brown sugar, cinnamon, and walnuts.
- Put honey in measuring cup and warm (either in microwave or water bath) until it flows easily.
- Drizzle the honey over the dry ingredients and mix to combine.
- Spread the mixture on a baking sheet lined with nonstick foil.
- Bake granola until golden and crunchy, stirring once, anywhere from 15 to 25 minutes.
- Stir in the raisins and flaxseed meal. Makes about 3 cups. Each serving is 3/4 cup.

Nutrition Facts   Nutrition (per serving): 358.0 calories; 18% calories from fat; 8.1g total fat; 0.0mg cholesterol; 8.7mg sodium; 332.9mg potassium; 71.5g carbohydrates; 7.8g fiber; 37.2g sugar; 7.5g protein.

Healthy Baked Garlic Tortilla Chips

Serves 2

2 whole wheat tortillas (pre-packaged)
1/4 tsp olive oil
2 cloves garlic, chopped

- Preheat oven to 450 degrees.
- Brush tortilla with olive oil.
- Bake in oven for one minute, until the tortilla just starts to bubble and become slightly brown, then remove.
- Brush with crushed garlic.

- Put back in oven and bake for another minute, until slightly toasted.
- Remove from oven, cut into 8 triangular pieces (like a pizza).

Nutrition Facts   Nutrition (per serving): 118.6 calories; 24% calories from fat; 3.3g total fat; 0.0mg cholesterol; 223.1mg sodium; 66.3mg potassium; 19.0g carbohydrates; 1.1g fiber; 0.7g sugar; 3.1g protein.

Horseradish Sauce

Serves 4

1 tsp horseradish (commercially prepared), white
1/4 cup sour cream, nonfat
1 tsp onion, chopped
1 tsp Worcestershire sauce
dash salt

- Mix above ingredients.

Nutrition Facts   Nutrition (per serving): 22.4 calories; 71% calories from fat; 1.8g total fat; 5.9mg cholesterol; 61.2mg sodium; 33.8mg potassium; 1.1g carbohydrates; 0.1g fiber; 0.2g sugar; 0.5g protein.

Hummus

Serves 4

1 tsp flaxseed meal
1/4 cup walnuts
1 can (19 oz) chickpeas
2 tbs fresh lemon juice
1/4 cup onions
2 cloves garlic
2 tsps flaxseed oil
2 tsps cumin powder
1/8 tsp red pepper flakes
1/2 tsp salt

- Drain chickpeas and save liquid.
- In food processor, place walnuts and flax meal. Chop until fine.

- Put garlic into walnut and flaxseed meal mixture and run food processor until garlic is chopped.
- Add cumin, lemon juice, onions, chickpeas and flaxseed oil to garlic, walnuts, and flax meal mixture in the food processor.
- Blend until smooth.
- Add reserved chickpea liquid, to thin to taste.
- Add red pepper flakes and salt to taste.
- Final product should be a semi-thick paste.

Nutrition Facts   Nutrition (per serving): 163.6 calories; 44% calories from fat; 8.6g total fat; 0.0mg cholesterol; 476.3mg sodium; 235.6mg potassium; 18.0g carbohydrates; 4.0g fiber; 0.8g sugar; 5.8g protein.

London Broil and Vegetable Wrap

Serves 1

1 whole wheat tortilla
1/4 cup chopped onion
1/4 cup cucumbers, chopped
1/2 cup chopped cabbage
1 serving London Broil, with garlic and ginger recipe, shredded
2 tbs Horseradish Sauce (see recipe)

- Combine onion, cabbage, cucumber, and shredded London Broil.
- Spread down the middle of the tortilla.
- Spoon one tablespoon of horseradish sauce over London Broil and vegetable mixture.
- Fold tortilla.

Nutrition Facts   Nutrition (per serving): 407.7 calories; 29% calories from fat; 13.2g total fat; 56.0mg cholesterol; 529.5mg sodium; 808.0mg potassium; 36.1g carbohydrates; 5.0g fiber; 4.0g sugar; 37.5g protein.

London Broil with Garlic Marinade

Serves 4

1 pound flank steak
Marinade

2 tbs Worcestershire sauce
1 tbs soy sauce
4 cloves garlic, chopped
1 dash cayenne pepper
1/4 tsp fresh ginger, chopped

- Combine all ingredients and marinate flank steak for at least two hours.
- Broil steak for about 7 minutes per side (until medium rare).
- Remove from oven and let rest for 10 minutes.
- Thinly slice against the grain.
- Serve with horseradish sauce.

Nutrition Facts   Nutrition (per serving): 216.4 calories; 34% calories from fat; 8.1g total fat; 44.2mg cholesterol; 391.2mg sodium; 481.0mg potassium; 2.6g carbohydrates; 0.1g fiber; 0.1g sugar; 32.3g protein.

Lox-Smoked Salmon or Nova

Serves 1

2 oz smoked nova salmon

Nutrition Facts   Nutrition (per serving): 66.3 calories; 33% calories from fat; 2.4g total fat; 13.0mg cholesterol; 1134.0mg sodium; 99.2mg potassium; 0.0g carbohydrates; 0.0g fiber; 0.0g sugar; 10.4g protein.

Macadamia Nut Encrusted Mahi-Mahi

Serves 2

1 tsp rice wine vinegar
1/2 tsp walnut oil
3/4 tsp pepper
1/4 tsp salt
2 Mahi-Mahi steaks (6 oz each – approximately 1-inch thick)
1/4 cup macadamia nuts, crushed

- Combine vinegar, oil, and spices.
- Brush oil mixture evenly over both sides of Mahi-Mahi steaks. Arrange Mahi-Mahi on oiled sheet pans.

- Place pans in preheated 425 degree oven. Cook approximately 5 minutes on each side, until fish flakes easily and reaches 145 degrees.
- Remove from the oven.
- Divide the crushed nuts among the tops of the 2 fillets, patting the mixture to spread and adhere to the fillets.
- Return to the oven and bake for 5 to 10 minutes, or until the crust is golden brown.
- Remove from the oven and allow to stand 10 minutes before serving.

Nutrition Facts   Nutrition (per serving): 222.6 calories; 54% calories from fat; 14.5g total fat; 38.3mg cholesterol; 323.3mg sodium; 465.1mg potassium; 3.8g carbohydrates; 1.5g fiber; 0.7g sugar; 21.2g protein.

Margaux's Mango and Banana Smoothie

Serves 2

1 banana
1/2 cup mango
1/2 cup 2% milk
1 tbs flaxseed oil
3 ice cubes

- Combine all ingredients into a blender.
- Mix until smooth.

Nutrition Facts   Nutrition (per serving): 173.1 calories; 39% calories from fat; 7.7g total fat; 3.0mg cholesterol; 29.7mg sodium; 399.7mg potassium; 25.6g carbohydrates; 2.5g fiber; 17.6g sugar; 3.0g protein.

Mary's Old-Fashioned Muesli with Dried Fruit

Serves 2

1/2 cup rolled oats
1/2 cup barley flakes
1 oz walnuts, chopped
1 oz almonds
1/2 oz dried cherries

1/2 oz dried cranberries
1 tbs flaxseed meal

- Put the oats into a bowl and stir in the remaining ingredients until evenly mixed. Store in an airtight container.

Nutrition Facts   Nutrition (per serving): 363.9 calories; 42% calories from fat; 18.7g total fat; 0.0mg cholesterol; 67.8mg sodium; 228.1mg potassium; 46.0g carbohydrates; 7.2g fiber; 3.3g sugar; 7.7g protein.

Mashed Sweet Potatoes and Spinach

Serves 4

4 sweet potatoes
2 cups spinach
3 cloves garlic
2 tbs olive oil

- Peel and boil potatoes until tender.
- Clean and chop spinach.
- Chop garlic and sauté in large pot until fragrant.
- Add spinach and sauté until wilted.
- Drain potatoes and mash into pot with spinach.

Nutrition Facts   Nutrition (per serving): 347.9 calories; 18% calories from fat; 7.2g total fat; 0.0mg cholesterol; 67.0mg sodium; 1848.4mg potassium; 69.8g carbohydrates; 0.4g fiber; 0.1g sugar; 6.2g protein.

Melanie's Mango and Avocado Salad with Pomegranate Vinaigrette Dressing

Serves 4

2 avocados
1 mango
Dressing:
2 tbs flaxseed oil
1 1/2 tbs pomegranate concentrate
2 tbs red wine vinegar

- Arrange sliced mango and avocado, alternating slices of each on single salad plate.
- Whisk flaxseed oil, pomegranate concentrate, and red wine vinegar.
- Drizzle dressing over mango and avocado.

Nutrition Facts   Nutrition (per serving): 263.2 calories; 65% calories from fat; 20.3g total fat; 0.0mg cholesterol; 8.2mg sodium; 526.8mg potassium; 22.5g carbohydrates; 6.8g fiber; 13.7g sugar; 2.2g protein.

Mixed Berries with Yogurt and Almonds
Serves 2

1/4 cup blueberries
1/4 cup raspberries
1/4 cup blackberries
2 tbs almonds, sliced
1 cup nonfat yogurt, plain
1 tsp flaxseed meal

- Fold berries, flaxseed meal, and almonds into yogurt.

Nutrition Facts   Nutrition (per serving): 160.3 calories; 37% calories from fat; 7.1g total fat; 7.5mg cholesterol; 86.6mg sodium; 417.4mg potassium; 16.9g carbohydrates; 3.7g fiber; 3.8g sugar; 9.2g protein.

Multigrain Cheerios with Fruit and Nuts
Serves 1

1 cup Multigrain Cheerios
1/4 cup blueberries
1 banana, sliced
1 tbs walnuts, chopped
1 tbs flaxseed meal

- Combine blueberries, bananas, and chopped walnuts with Cheerios.
- Sprinkle flaxseed meal over cereal.

Nutrition Facts   Nutrition (per serving): 317.1 calories; 22% calories from fat; 8.7g total fat; 0.0mg cholesterol; 255.8mg sodium; 581.2mg potassium; 59.8g carbohydrates; 8.4g fiber; 24.6g sugar; 6.8g protein.

Mustard Salmon

Serves 4

4 (3 oz) salmon steaks, wild (not farm-raised)
2 tbs Dijon mustard
1/2 tbs fresh thyme, finely chopped
1 tsp turmeric
2 tbs fresh lemon juice

- Combine mustard, thyme, turmeric, and lemon juice.
- Brush onto salmon and refrigerate for one hour.
- Preheat oven at 420 degrees.
- Cook salmon until done, about 20 minutes.

Nutrition Facts   Nutrition (per serving): 130.5 calories; 39% calories from fat; 5.8g total fat; 46.8mg cholesterol; 131.6mg sodium; 451.4mg potassium; 1.6g carbohydrates; 0.4g fiber; 0.2g sugar; 17.3g protein.

Omega Oatmeal

Serves 1

1/2 cup Quaker Whole Grain Oatmeal
1/4 teaspoon cinnamon
1 tbs flaxseed meal
1/4 cup dried cherries
1 cup water

- Combine water, oatmeal, cinnamon, and dried cherries.
- Microwave for 2 to 3 minutes.
- Remove from microwave.
- Add flaxseed meal and stir.

Nutrition Facts   Nutrition (per serving): 299.9 calories; 15% calories from fat; 5.5g total fat; 0.0mg cholesterol; 13.4mg sodium; 148.4mg potassium; 59.7g carbohydrates; 8.1g fiber; 0.6g sugar; 8.0g protein.

Orange and Pomegranate Juice

Serves 1

6 oz fresh orange juice
2 tbs pomegranate concentrate
1 tbs flaxseed oil

- Pour pomegranate concentrate into glass.
- Pour orange juice into glass.
- Add flaxseed oil.
- Mix.

Nutrition Facts   Nutrition (per serving): 331.4 calories; 37% calories from fat; 14.0g total fat; 0.0mg cholesterol; 2.6mg sodium; 372.0mg potassium; 50.1g carbohydrates; 0.4g fiber; 46.4g sugar; 2.8g protein.

Panko Chicken with Black Cherry Sauce

Serves 2

2 chicken breast halves (boneless, skin removed)
1/4 cup Panko
2 tbs flaxseed meal
1 tbs garlic powder
1 tbs oregano
1 tbs basil
4 tbs Black Cherry Sauce (see recipe)

- Combine Panko whole wheat bread crumbs, garlic powder, oregano, flaxseed meal, and basil.
- Pat onto chicken breast halves.
- Preheat oven to 450 degrees.
- Bake chicken for 40 minutes, or until done.
- Heat black cherry sauce and spoon two tablespoons on each chicken breast.

Nutrition Facts   Nutrition (per serving): 232.4 calories; 14% calories from fat; 3.9g total fat; 68.4mg cholesterol; 109.3mg sodium; 430.6mg potassium; 18.7g carbohydrates; 3.2g fiber; 10.2g sugar; 30.2g protein.

Portabella Mushrooms Stuffed with Crab

Serves 2

4 portabella mushrooms
2 cans (6.5 oz each) lump crab meat
1 tbs fresh lemon juice
1 tsp walnut oil
1 tbs yellow pepper, finely chopped
2 tbs shallots, finely chopped
2 tbs onions
3 cloves garlic, finely chopped
1/4 tsp cumin powder
1/4 tsp dry mustard
2 tsp Worcestershire sauce
1/4 tsp tarragon
1 tsp paprika
2 tbs fresh parsley, finely chopped

- Preheat the oven to 375 degrees.
- Arrange the portabellas on an oiled, ovenproof baking dish.
- Squeeze the lemon juice over the crab and toss very gently.
- In a small skillet, heat walnut oil and cook the peppers, onion, garlic, and shallots until tender.
- Remove from the heat and set aside.
- Stir into the cooked vegetable mixture the dry mustard, Worcestershire, tarragon, and cumin.
- Fold lump crabmeat into the vegetable mixture.
- Spoon the crab mixture into the portabella mushrooms.
- Bake in the preheated oven for 30 to 35 minutes or until top is brown.
- Sprinkle lightly with paprika and freshly chopped parsley.

Nutrition Facts   Nutrition (per serving): 258.4 calories; 16% calories from fat; 4.8g total fat; 111.3mg cholesterol; 490.1mg sodium; 2201.5mg potassium; 23.2g carbohydrates; 5.7g fiber; 6.6g sugar; 34.9g protein.

Power Tomato Juice

Serves 1

8 oz tomato juice (low sodium)
1 tbs flaxseed oil
dash Tabasco sauce

- Combine cold tomato juice, flaxseed oil, and Tabasco sauce in glass.
- Stir well.

Nutrition Facts Nutrition (per serving): 170.2 calories; 71% calories from fat; 13.8g total fat; 0.0mg cholesterol; 161.7mg sodium; 438.3mg potassium; 10.4g carbohydrates; 1.8g fiber; 8.6g sugar; 1.4g protein.

Raisins and Brown Rice

Serves 2

1 cup brown rice
2 cups water
1/4 cup raisins
1 tsp cinnamon
1 tsp turmeric

- Put rice, cinnamon, turmeric, raisins, and water into a medium-sized pot.
- Bring to a boil and then cover with a tight-fitting lid. Reduce heat and let simmer until rice has absorbed all of the liquid and is tender, about 30 minutes.

Nutrition Facts Nutrition (per serving): 178.8 calories; 5% calories from fat; 1.1g total fat; 0.0mg cholesterol; 15.1mg sodium; 215.8mg potassium; 41.4g carbohydrates; 4.4g fiber; 12.6g sugar; 3.3g protein.

Raspberry, Pomegranate, and Ginger Topping

Serves 6

1 cup raspberries
1 tbs pomegranate concentrate

1/4 tsp fresh ginger, chopped
1 dash cayenne pepper
1/2 tsp honey

- Put all ingredients into a blender.
- Strain with colander to remove seeds.
- Store in refrigerator in sealed plastic container.

Nutrition Facts   Nutrition (per serving): 26.1 calories; 5% calories from fat; 0.2g total fat; 0.0mg cholesterol; 0.4mg sodium; 40.5mg potassium; 6.2g carbohydrates; 1.7g fiber; 4.2g sugar; 0.4g protein.

Ricotta and Blueberry Parfait

Serves 1

1/2 cup ricotta cheese
1/4 cup blueberries
1/4 tsp vanilla

- Add vanilla to ricotta cheese.
- Use parfait glass and layer blueberries alternating with ricotta cheese.

Nutrition Facts   Nutrition (per serving): 238.1 calories; 59% calories from fat; 16.1g total fat; 62.7mg cholesterol; 103.8mg sodium; 159.2mg potassium; 9.2g carbohydrates; 0.9g fiber; 4.2g sugar; 14.1g protein.

Roasted Asparagus

Serves 4

1 pound asparagus
1/4 tbs walnut oil
1/2 tsp salt
1 tsp flaxseed meal

- Preheat oven to 425 degrees.
- Cut off the woody bottom part of the asparagus spears and discard.
- Use a vegetable peeler to peel off the skin on the bottom 2–3" of the spears.

- Place asparagus, walnut oil, and salt in a plastic baggie and mix until asparagus are coated with oil and salt.
- Place asparagus on foil-lined baking sheet and roast for 10 to 15 minutes or until tender.
- Remove from oven, sprinkle flaxseed meal over asparagus.

Nutrition Facts   Nutrition (per serving): 45.9 calories; 38% calories from fat; 2.0g total fat; 0.0mg cholesterol; 293.0mg sodium; 229.1mg potassium; 4.6g carbohydrates; 2.5g fiber; 2.1g sugar; 2.6g protein.

Salad with Ginger Dressing
Serves 1

1 cup iceberg lettuce, shredded
1/2 cup chopped scallion
1 medium tomato
1/4 tsp sesame seeds, toasted
1 tbs Ginger Dressing (see recipe)

- Chop lettuce and scallion, place in a bowl.
- Cut tomato in half and squeeze out seeds and juice, cut out pulp, and slice in thin strips.
- Toss ginger dressing with lettuce, tomato, and scallion.
- Sprinkle with sesame seeds.

Nutrition Facts   Nutrition (per serving): 83.8 calories; 38% calories from fat; 4.2g total fat; 0.0mg cholesterol; 276.3mg sodium; 547.3mg potassium; 12.1g carbohydrates; 3.4g fiber; 4.8g sugar; 3.2g protein.

Salmon with Ginger-Orange Sauce
Serves 2

2 wild salmon fillets
3 tsp fresh ginger, grated
2 cloves garlic
1 tbs orange juice
1 tsp Tamari sauce

1 tsp walnut oil
1 tsp curry powder

- Preheat oven to 400 degrees.
- In a food processor, blend walnut oil, ginger, garlic, orange juice, tamari sauce, and curry powder.
- Brush salmon fillets evenly with ginger mixture.
- Place in a medium baking dish.
- Bake 15 to 20 minutes in the preheated oven, until the fish flakes easily with a fork.

Nutrition Facts   Nutrition (per serving): 156.0 calories; 44% calories from fat; 7.8g total fat; 46.8mg cholesterol; 206.5mg sodium; 478.3mg potassium; 3.1g carbohydrates; 0.5g fiber; 0.8g sugar; 17.6g protein.

Sautéed Broccoli Rabe

Serves 4

1 head broccoli rabe, trimmed and washed
5 tbs walnut oil
1 clove garlic, minced
1 tbs parmesan, grated

- Bring large pot of salted water to a boil.
- Cut an X in bottom of stems of broccoli rabe and place in boiling water.
- Cook 5 minutes, then drain in colander.
- In a large skillet over medium heat, sauté garlic in oil 1 to 2 minutes.
- Stir in rabe and sauté 10 to15 minutes more or until firm but tender.
- Dust with parmesan cheese and serve immediately.

Nutrition Facts   Nutrition (per serving): 188.5 calories; 83% calories from fat; 17.8g total fat; 1.1mg cholesterol; 316.3mg sodium; 336.8mg potassium; 6.0g carbohydrates; 3.8g fiber; 1.6g sugar; 3.9g protein.

Sautéed Kale with Garlic and Mushrooms

Serves 2

1 cup kale
1/2 cup white mushrooms, sliced
2 cloves garlic, minced
1/2 tsp olive oil

- Boil kale until cooked, then drain.
- In pan, heat olive oil and sauté garlic.
- Add mushrooms and cook until tender.
- Add kale to mushrooms and garlic and mix.

Nutrition Facts   Nutrition (per serving): 35.0 calories; 35% calories from fat; 1.4g total fat; 0.0mg cholesterol; 15.8mg sodium; 217.4mg potassium; 4.9g carbohydrates; 0.9g fiber; 0.3g sugar; 1.8g protein.

Scrambled Egg Whites Italiano

Serves 1

4 large egg whites
3 baby portabellas (crimini), diced
2 tsp olive oil
1/4 tsp turmeric
1/4 tsp fresh oregano, chopped
1/4 tsp fresh basil, chopped
2 tsp 1% milk
1 tsp flaxseed meal
1 dash salt

- Put egg whites into mixing bowl. Beat slightly using wire whisk.
- Add milk, turmeric, oregano, basil, flaxseed meal, and salt to eggs. Beat until blended.
- Heat olive oil in frying pan. Add mushrooms, and cook until soft.
- Pour in egg mixture. Cook over low heat, stirring occasionally, until reaching desired consistency.

Nutrition Facts   Nutrition (per serving): 177.1 calories; 50% calories from fat; 10.2g total fat; 0.5mg cholesterol; 384.2mg sodium; 438.4mg potassium; 4.3g carbohydrates; 1.1g fiber; 2.2g sugar; 16.5g protein.

Scrambled Eggs with Onions, Green Peppers

Serves 1

1/2 cup egg whites (approx. 4 eggs)
1/2 tbs walnut oil
3 tbs onion, diced
1 clove garlic, finely chopped
3 tbs diced green bell pepper
1 dash black pepper
1/4 tsp turmeric
2 oz water

- Heat walnut oil in a nonstick pan.
- Sauté green pepper, garlic, pepper, and onions for about 2 minutes.
- Whisk turmeric and water into egg whites.
- Add egg mixture to pepper and onions, cook until firm.

Nutrition Facts   Nutrition (per serving): 189.8 calories; 51% calories from fat; 11.1g total fat; 1.3mg cholesterol; 224.9mg sodium; 534.0mg potassium; 6.3g carbohydrates; 1.2g fiber; 2.8g sugar; 15.9g protein.

Seafood Salad

Serves 2

12 shrimp, deveined, cleaned and cooked with tails removed
3 oz crabmeat, canned, drained
1/4 head iceberg lettuce, shredded
1 medium cucumber, chopped
1/4 cup onion, chopped
6 cherry tomatoes
1 carrot, chopped
1 stalk celery, chopped
2 tbs Special Balsamic Vinaigrette Dressing (see recipe)

- Combine shrimp, lettuce, cucumber, onion, carrot, celery, and tomatoes in a bowl. Toss with dressing.
- Top with crabmeat.

Nutrition Facts   Nutrition (per serving): 180.3 calories; 35% calories from fat; 7.3g total fat; 89.4mg cholesterol; 262.4mg sodium; 761.2mg potassium; 12.8g carbohydrates; 3.6g fiber; 4.7g sugar; 16.7g protein.

Seafood Stew

Serves 4

4 tbs walnut oil
1 large onion, chopped
3 scallions, chopped
4 cloves garlic, chopped
1 medium tomato, chopped
2 tbs tomato paste
8 oz clam juice
1/4 pound shrimp, cleaned, deveined, tails removed
1 pound cod
1/4 pound scallops
1 tbs fresh basil
1 tbs fresh parsley
1 tbs fresh thyme
1 tbs fresh cilantro
1 tbs fresh oregano
1 tsp paprika
1 tbs flaxseed meal

- Heat oil in heavy pot.
- Add onion, scallions, and garlic. Sauté over medium heat for about 5 minutes, until onion is soft. Do not brown garlic.
- Add parsley and cook for 2 minutes.
- Add basil, thyme, cilantro, oregano, paprika, clam juice, tomato, and tomato paste. Cook 2 minutes.
- Add cod and scallops and cook until tender.
- Add shrimp and cook until they turn pink.
- Remove from heat and add flaxseed meal.

Nutrition Facts   Nutrition (per serving): 388.3 calories; 42% calories from fat; 18.5g total fat; 114.7mg cholesterol; 551.9mg sodium; 964.3mg potassium; 20.8g carbohydrates; 2.9g fiber; 5.2g sugar; 34.9g protein.

Seared Tuna with Mango Salsa

Serves 4

4 tuna steaks
Marinade
1/4 cup fresh lime juice
1 tbs walnut oil
2 tbs tamari sauce
1/4 tsp mustard, dry
Salsa
1 mango, ripe, diced
1/4 cup scallions
2 tbs fresh cilantro
1 cucumber
1 clove garlic
1 tbs fresh lime juice
1 tsp fresh ginger, finely minced
1/2 tbs flaxseed oil
1/2 tsp kosher salt

For Marinade:
- Combine lime juice, walnut oil, tamari sauce, and dry mustard into a bowl and whisk.
- Pour marinade over tuna and refrigerate for a 1/2 hour.

For Mango Salsa:
- Finely chop mango, scallions, cucumber, garlic, and cilantro and combine in a bowl.
- Add lime juice, ginger, flaxseed oil, and salt to above, refrigerate.
- Sear tuna in frying pan about 5 minutes each side.
- Serve tuna on plate, spoon on salsa.

Nutrition Facts   Nutrition (per serving): 192.4 calories; 28% calories from fat; 6.2g total fat; 38.3mg cholesterol; 829.9mg sodium; 607.2mg potassium; 13.1g carbohydrates; 1.7g fiber; 9.0g sugar; 21.7g protein.

Sesame Snow Peas with Basil

Serves 4

1 lb snow peas
3 tbs toasted sesame seeds
1 tsp flax oil
2 tbs fresh basil, chopped
1 tbs flax meal

- Trim the stem end of the peas, remove string.
- Boil a pot of water and add peas.
- Blanch peas until they turn bright green, about 1 minute.
- Pour into strainer and shake dry.
- Pour peas into a bowl and add flax oil.
- Toss with toasted sesame seeds and flax meal.
- Sprinkle with basil and serve warm or chilled.

Nutrition Facts   Nutrition (per serving): 144.9 calories; 31% calories from fat; 5.4g total fat; 0.0mg cholesterol; 82.4mg sodium; 162.5mg potassium; 18.3g carbohydrates; 7.6g fiber; 5.3g sugar; 7.4g protein.

Sesame Tuna Steaks

Serves 1

1 (3 oz) yellow fin tuna steak
1 tbs tamari sauce
1 tbs fresh ginger, minced
1 tbs sesame seeds
1 tsp fresh cilantro, chopped
1 tbs canola oil

- Combine tamari sauce, ginger, cilantro, and sesame seeds.
- Brush onto tuna fillets.
- Refrigerate for one hour.
- Heat oil in frying pan.
- Sear tuna on each side for about 2 minutes.

Nutrition Facts   Nutrition (per serving): 283.1 calories; 59% calories from fat; 19.3g total fat; 38.3mg cholesterol; 1039.6mg sodium; 490.7mg potassium; 4.2g carbohydrates; 1.4g fiber; 0.4g sugar; 23.5g protein.

Shrimp and Garlic in Lime Juice

Serves 4

1 1/2 lb shrimp, cleaned, deveined with
shells and tails removed
5 limes (juiced)
1 lemon (juiced)
5 cloves garlic, minced
5 tbs fresh cilantro, chopped
1 tsp brown sugar
1 tsp olive oil
6 oz snow peas

- Combine lime juice, lemon juice, garlic, cilantro, brown sugar, and oil.
- Add shrimp and marinate in the refrigerator for 1/2 hour.
- Heat frying pan and add marinated shrimp and snow peas.
- Cook until shrimp turns pink.

Nutrition Facts Nutrition (per serving): 236.9 calories; 15% calories from fat; 4.2g total fat; 258.6mg cholesterol; 259.0mg sodium; 532.0mg potassium; 13.3g carbohydrates; 1.6g fiber; 4.1g sugar; 36.4g protein.

Sliced Peach with Raspberry, Pomegranate, and Ginger Topping

Serves 1

1 fresh peach, sliced
1 tbs Raspberry, Pomegranate, and Ginger Topping

- Top fresh sliced peach with raspberry, pomegranate, and ginger topping.

Nutrition Facts Nutrition (per serving): 83.4 calories; 5% calories from fat; 0.5g total fat; 0.0mg cholesterol; 0.4mg sodium; 319.8mg potassium; 20.2g carbohydrates; 3.9g fiber; 16.5g sugar; 1.8g protein.

Sol's Salmon with Horseradish and Ginger Panko Crust

Serves 4

4 (3 oz) wild salmon fillets, skin removed
1/2 cup Panko whole wheat bread crumbs
2 tbs prepared horseradish, white, drained of liquid
4 tsp flaxseed meal
2 tsp ginger, fresh grated
2 tbs fresh lemon juice
1 tbs olive oil
1/4 tsp salt
1/4 tsp pepper

- Put Panko bread crumbs into food processor and process until finely chopped.
- Add horseradish, flaxseed meal, ginger, lemon juice, salt, pepper, and olive oil to bread crumbs. Process until smooth.
- Press bread crumb mixture onto salmon fillets.
- Broil for about 8 minutes, until crust is brown.

Nutrition Facts   Nutrition (per serving): 186.7 calories; 45% calories from fat; 9.6g total fat; 46.8mg cholesterol; 215.1mg sodium; 450.3mg potassium; 6.4g carbohydrates; 1.2g fiber; 3.3g sugar; 18.0g protein.

Spanish Garlic Soup

Serves 6

5 cups vegetable broth
10 cloves garlic, peeled and sliced
1 cup dry sherry
1/4 cup olive oil
1 tbs parmesan cheese, fat free
salt to taste
pepper to taste
6 whole wheat bread slices

- Sauté garlic in the oil until it turns golden.

- Heat the broth and sherry until it boils and then add the cooked garlic and olive oil.
- Season with salt and pepper to taste and simmer 30 minutes.
- Strain out the garlic and reheat.
- Sprinkle toasted bread slices with the cheese, then place them in a 425 degree oven for 3 minutes.
- Put the toast in the bottom of soup dishes; pour the soup over the top.
- Serve immediately.

Nutrition Facts   Nutrition (per serving): 311.9 calories; 31% calories from fat; 11.2g total fat; 3.3mg cholesterol; 416.2mg sodium; 540.3mg potassium; 34.3g carbohydrates; 5.0g fiber; 6.8g sugar; 12.6g protein.

Special Balsamic Vinaigrette Dressing

Serves 12

1/3 cup flax oil
1/3 cup balsamic vinegar
3 cloves garlic, chopped
1 dash cayenne pepper

- Combine all ingredients in a bowl and whisk.
- Keep refrigerated.

Nutrition Facts   Nutrition (per serving): 55.2 calories; 94% calories from fat; 6.0g total fat; 0.0mg cholesterol; 0.3mg sodium; 10.6mg potassium; 0.7g carbohydrates; 0.0g fiber; 0.0g sugar; 0.0g protein.

Spiced Twice Baked Sweet Potato

Serves 1

1 sweet potato
1/4 tsp walnut oil
1 pat butter
cinnamon to taste

- Scrub sweet potato; brush with walnut oil.
- Bake at 450 degrees for 35 to 45 minutes, or until tender.

- Remove at once and prick with a fork to let steam out. Cut potato in half and shell out sweet potato, leaving the skin.
- Mix potato with butter and cinnamon. Put back into skin.
- Bake at 450 degrees for another 10 minutes.

Nutrition Facts   Nutrition (per serving): 207.8 calories; 23% calories from fat; 5.5g total fat; 10.8mg cholesterol; 65.3mg sodium; 856.2mg potassium; 37.3g carbohydrates; 5.9g fiber; 11.7g sugar; 3.7g protein.

Spicy Garlic and Ginger Chicken

Serves 4

2 to 3 lb chicken (free-range), white meat

1 tsp lite soy sauce

1 tsp white wine

1 tsp cornstarch

1 tbs garlic, minced

1 tbs fresh cilantro root

10 slices ginger

1 1/2 tbs fish sauce

1 1/2 tbs soy sauce

2 tbs walnut oil

1/2 tsp sugar

1 tsp pepper

2 tbs water

- Cut chicken into strips.
- Marinate chicken with the lite soy sauce, wine, and cornstarch.
- Heat 2 tablespoons of walnut oil and stir-fry garlic, cilantro and ginger until fragrant.
- Add chicken and stir-fry until cooked.
- Add fish sauce, sweet soy sauce, sugar, and pepper. Mix well.
- Add water and bring to a boil.
- Serve.

Nutrition Facts   Nutrition (per serving): 106.2 calories; 9% calories from fat; 1.0g total fat; 44.1mg cholesterol; 994.1mg sodium; 276.9mg potassium; 4.1g carbohydrates; 0.4g fiber; 1.0g sugar; 19.0g protein.

Spinach and Garlic

Serves 2

2 cups spinach
2 cloves garlic, minced
1/2 tsp olive oil

- Boil spinach and drain.
- In pan, heat olive oil and sauté garlic.
- Add spinach to garlic and mix.

Nutrition Facts   Nutrition (per serving): 21.3 calories; 51% calories from fat; 1.3g total fat; 0.0mg cholesterol; 24.2mg sodium; 179.4mg potassium; 2.1g carbohydrates; 0.7g fiber; 0.2g sugar; 1.0g protein.

Stonyfield Farm Vanilla Nonfat Frozen Yogurt

Serves 1

1/2 cup frozen yogurt, soft serve

Nutrition Facts   Nutrition (per serving): 100.0 calories; 0% calories from fat; 0.0g total fat; 7.0mg cholesterol; 70.0mg sodium; 220.0mg potassium; 21.0g carbohydrates; 0.0g fiber; 19.0g sugar; 4.0g protein.

Sweet Potato and Leek Soup

Serves 4

2 leeks, white and light green parts washed well (all sand removed)
and cut into 1/4-inch slices
2 cups red onions, chopped
3 cloves garlic, minced
2 sweet potatoes, peeled and cubed into 1/2-inch cubes
2 large carrots, cut into 1/2 rounds
4 cups vegetable stock
nonstick vegetable spray
1/2 teaspoon ground cumin seed
1 teaspoon flaxseed meal

- Heat a 4-quart soup pot over medium heat and spray with vegetable spray.
- Add the carrots and sauté until slightly soft.
- Add the garlic and stir well. Cook for 1 minute more.
- Add leeks and onions. Sauté for about 5 minutes, stirring often, until the onion begins to turn translucent.
- Add cumin, potatoes, and vegetable stock, cover, and bring to a boil.
- Reduce heat to simmer. Cook 20 minutes.
- Remove the soup from the heat.
- Blend the soup in a food processor until smooth.
- Strain soup through fine colander or chinois into a pot and warm over low heat.
- Stir in flaxseed meal.
- You can freeze extra soup in serving-sized containers.

Nutrition Facts   Nutrition (per serving): 99.7 calories; 6% calories from fat; 0.8g total fat; 0.0mg cholesterol; 597.0mg sodium; 234.5mg potassium; 20.8g carbohydrates; 27.9g fiber; 1.1g sugar; 2.7g protein.

Sweet Potato Hash

Serves 4

1 sweet potato, diced
2 tbs walnut oil
1/2 cup red onions, diced
1 tsp cumin powder
1/4 cup pecans, chopped
1/2 cup parsley, chopped

- Preheat a large nonstick skillet over medium high heat with 2 table-spoons of walnut oil.
- Dice sweet potato into 1/4-inch cubes.
- Add the sweet potato, diced red onion, and cumin. Stir frequently and cook for 10 to 12 minutes, or until the potato is tender.
- Add pecans and stir for one minute.
- Put on plate and sprinkle parsley over dish.

Nutrition Facts   Nutrition (per serving): 146.6 calories; 70% calories from fat; 11.9g total fat; 0.0mg cholesterol; 23.5mg sodium; 188.4mg potassium; 9.7g carbohydrates; 2.3g fiber; 1.7g sugar; 1.7g protein.

Tarragon Lamb Chops

Serves 1

2 lamb chops (loin)
2 cloves garlic, chopped
1/2 tsp tarragon
1/4 tsp turmeric

- Season lamb chops with tarragon, garlic, and turmeric.
- Broil until cooked as desired.

Nutrition Facts   Nutrition (per serving): 132.6 calories; 34% calories from fat; 5.1g total fat; 68.4mg cholesterol; 34.7mg sodium; 175.5mg potassium; 2.7g carbohydrates; 0.3g fiber; 0.1g sugar; 18.2g protein.

Three Spice Baked Chicken

Serves 4

4 free-range chicken breast pieces, boneless and skinless
1 tbs walnut oil
3/4 tsp cumin, ground
1/4 tsp fresh thyme
1/2 tsp fresh sage, finely chopped
2 cloves garlic, finely chopped
1/4 tsp salt
1/2 tsp pepper

- Preheat oven to 375 degrees.
- Clean chicken and pat dry.
- Brush chicken with walnut oil.
- Mix salt, thyme, sage, cumin, garlic, and pepper in a bowl.
- On large, greased baking pan with sides, place chicken. Pat seasonings mixture onto the chicken breasts.

- Place in 375 degree oven and cook about 20 minutes or until meat is no longer pink when tested with a knife.

Nutrition Facts   Nutrition (per serving): 154.5 calories; 22% calories from fat; 3.8g total fat; 68.4mg cholesterol; 245.6mg sodium; 318.2mg potassium; 0.9g carbohydrates; 0.2g fiber; 0.0g sugar; 27.5g protein.

Tossed Salad with Special Balsamic Vinaigrette Dressing
Serves 2

1/4 head lettuce (of your choice) shredded
1 tomato, sliced
1/4 cup red onions, chopped
1/4 cup red sweet pepper, chopped
1/4 cup carrots, grated
1 tsp flaxseed meal
2 tbs Special Balsamic Vinaigrette Dressing (see recipe)

- Combine all ingredients in a bowl and toss with dressing.

Nutrition Facts   Nutrition (per serving): 91.0 calories; 63% calories from fat; 6.6g total fat; 0.0mg cholesterol; 25.5mg sodium; 283.9mg potassium; 7.8g carbohydrates; 2.4g fiber; 3.5g sugar; 1.7g protein.

Tropical Fruit Salad
Serves 2

1 cup mango, diced
1/2 cup papaya, diced
1 cup pineapple, chopped
1/2 cup cherries, pitted and chopped
1 cup blueberries
1 banana, sliced
1/4 cup walnuts, chopped

- Mix all ingredients and enjoy.

Nutrition Facts   Nutrition (per serving): 324.5 calories; 27% calories from fat; 10.5g total fat; 0.0mg cholesterol; 6.6mg sodium; 775.1mg potassium; 60.8g carbohydrates; 8.5g fiber; 41.0g sugar; 5.0g protein.

Turkey Meatloaf

Serves 6

2 lbs ground turkey
1/2 cup Panko whole wheat bread crumbs
2 egg whites
3/4 cup fat-free milk
1/2 cup Vidalia onions
1/2 tsp salt
1/2 tsp pepper
1 tsp fresh oregano, chopped
1 tsp fresh parsley, chopped
1 tsp minced garlic
1 tsp fresh basil, chopped
1/4 tsp mustard

- Preheat oven to 350 degrees.
- In a large bowl, mix together all ingredients.
- When all ingredients are mixed, shape into a meatloaf.
- Put meatloaf into a baking pan.
- Bake at 350 degrees for 1 hour to 1 hour 15 minutes.

Nutrition Facts Nutrition (per serving): 275.4 calories; 41% calories from fat; 12.8g total fat; 120.1mg cholesterol; 473.1mg sodium; 607.9mg potassium; 8.6g carbohydrates; 1.1g fiber; 4.0g sugar; 30.0g protein.

Vegetable Stock

Serves 5

5 cups water
2 onions
2 carrots
2 celery stalks
2 leeks, well-cleaned (sand removed), chopped
1 bay leaf
1/2 cup parsley, chopped

- Peel and quarter onions.
- Wash and cut carrots into large pieces.
- Wash and cut celery (including leaves) into large pieces.
- Clean leeks (remove sand), cut into large pieces.
- Combine above ingredients and put in stockpot.
- Add bay leaf, parsley, and water to pot. Add more water if needed to cover vegetables.
- Bring to a boil, then simmer covered for one hour.
- Remove pot from stove and drain vegetables from broth using a colander or cheesecloth.

Nutrition Facts   Nutrition (per serving): 63.9 calories; 4% calories from fat; 0.3g total fat; 0.0mg cholesterol; 60.3mg sodium; 346.1mg potassium; 14.6g carbohydrates; 3.1g fiber; 5.8g sugar; 1.8g protein.

Veggie Frittata

Serves 4

1 tsp olive oil
1 cup egg whites (approx. 8 eggs)
1 cup onion, chopped
2 cups kale, chopped
2 cloves garlic, chopped
1/4 tsp turmeric
1 cup tomatoes, chopped
1 tbs parsley, chopped
4 oz water

- Heat nonstick oven-safe pan and add olive oil.
- Sauté onion and garlic.
- Add kale and cook until soft.
- Add tomatoes, stir and cook over low heat for about 2 minutes.
- Blend turmeric and water with egg whites.
- Pour egg whites over vegetable mixture, cover and cook over low heat until firm.
- Sprinkle parsley on top of egg mixture.

- Place pan in oven and broil for 3 to 4 minutes until the top is lightly brown.
- Remove from pan and serve immediately.

Nutrition Facts   Nutrition (per serving): 106.6 calories; 29% calories from fat; 3.6g total fat; 0.6mg cholesterol; 130.2mg sodium; 536.6mg potassium; 9.9g carbohydrates; 2.0g fiber; 3.3g sugar; 9.6g protein.

Very Veggie Chili
Serves 6

1 large onion, minced
1 clove garlic, minced
1 medium shallot, minced
3 large scallions, minced
1 large red or green pepper chopped
1 tsp olive oil
15 oz tomato sauce (low sodium)
15 oz canned tomatoes, chopped
19 oz can of kidney beans
1 tsp miso paste
1 tbs chili powder
1 tsp curry powder
1 tbs fresh basil, chopped
1 tsp ground cumin
salt and pepper

- In a large saucepan, sauté onion, shallot, garlic, scallions, and pepper in olive oil.
- Add tomato sauce, chopped canned tomatoes, miso paste, and spices. Cook on low for 1 hour, occasionally stirring.
- Add kidney beans. Cook until beans are tender.
- Salt and pepper to taste.
- Serve over brown rice, if desired.

Nutrition Facts   Nutrition (per serving): 209.3 calories; 7% calories from fat; 1.9g total fat; 0.0mg cholesterol; 424.7mg sodium; 1025.8mg potassium; 41.4g carbohydrates; 10.3g fiber; 6.2g sugar; 9.8g protein.

Whole Grain Cheerios with Flax Meal

Serves 1

1 cup Whole Grain Cheerios
1 tbs flaxseed meal

- Sprinkle flaxseed meal over Cheerios.

Nutrition Facts   Nutrition (per serving): 141.9 calories; 19% calories from fat; 3.3g total fat; 0.0mg cholesterol; 254.1mg sodium; 97.2mg potassium; 26.5g carbohydrates; 3.9g fiber; 6.3g sugar; 4.1g protein.

Yellow Squash with Lemon

Serves 2

2 tbs walnut oil
1/2 cup onions
1 clove garlic, minced
1 yellow squash
3 plum tomatoes, chopped
2 tbs fresh lemon juice
salt and pepper

- Heat oil and cook onions until soft.
- Add garlic and cook for about one minute.
- Add chopped tomatoes, squash, and lemon juice. Cook until squash is soft (about 10 minutes).
- Salt and pepper to taste.

Nutrition Facts   Nutrition (per serving): 200.0 calories; 61% calories from fat; 13.9g total fat; 0.0mg cholesterol; 252.7mg sodium; 594.8mg potassium; 19.9g carbohydrates; 1.9g fiber; 6.5g sugar; 2.3g protein.

Yogurt Cinnamon and Nutmeg Topping

Serves 6

1/2 cup yogurt, low fat, vanilla
1 pinch cinnamon
1 pinch nutmeg

- Combine yogurt, cinnamon, and nutmeg.

Nutrition Facts   Nutrition (per serving): 18.6 calories; 13% calories from fat; 0.3g total fat; 1.0mg cholesterol; 13.6mg sodium; 46.8mg potassium; 3.1g carbohydrates; 0.2g fiber; 2.8g sugar; 1.0g protein.

10

Getting Help

DOCTORS WANT "GOOD" patients. By "good," they generally mean "cooperative." Why? Because cooperation equals successful results. Patients also want "good" doctors, by which they usually mean doctors who know what they're doing and have an empathetic bedside manner. Those qualities make patients feel safe, trusting, and cared for. Unfortunately, these attitudes on the part of both doctor and patient can lead to a relationship that locks the caregiver into an active role but leaves the recipient—you—in a passive one.

Medical treatment works best when physician and patient are full partners in care. For this to happen, your doctor needs to be generous with time and expertise, and you need to be knowledgeable about what realistically to expect from the diagnostic/therapeutic process—as well as how to make judgments along the way.

Your first decision? When to seek help.

Is Today the Day?

How do you know when it's time to see a doctor? Your body will give you signals. Listen to them. Consult a physician if you experience:

Sudden pain. This means severe joint pain that comes out of the blue, and/or you experience heat or swelling in or around a joint. Do NOT wait for a week or two to see if the pain, swelling, or heat goes away on its own.

Injury. It's especially important to make a medical appointment if you have a joint injury that results in severe pain. The more quickly and appropriately you treat an injury, the more likely you will be to make a complete recovery.

Fever or rash. If a fever or skin rash develops along with joint pain or swelling, you may be in the initial stages of RA, gout, or even an infection. It's especially important to treat this condition early, when controlling or even reversing the disease may be possible.

Persistent discomfort. Joint pain or swelling that lasts longer than one week, even if it's not severe, needs to be evaluated.

A poor score. If your ADQ score in chapter one was 16 or higher, I strongly recommend that you see a rheumatologist. A score at that level means your condition has progressed beyond the home treatment stage. I also recommend you see a doctor if your ADQ score was initially between 8 and 16 and has not decreased by at least 6 points after being on my program eight weeks, or if your score was initially between 0 and 7 and it has increased by any number.

MAKING LIFE A LITTLE EASIER

To protect your knees while weeding, kneel on a partially filled hot water bottle for cushioning.

The Best Person for the Job

Whom you go to for help depends upon what your symptoms are. Acute care may require one kind of doctor, whereas long-term care might require another. Here is who to see:

For an injury.   If you've suffered an injury, such as from an accident, a fall, or a sports mishap, you're best off going either to an orthopedist's office or a hospital emergency room as quickly as possible. Either will be prepared to give you emergency treatment for extreme conditions, such as a bone fracture.

For recent onset of joint pain.   Joint pain can have many causes. Your family doctor may be able to make an initial diagnosis and send you to an appropriate specialist, if necessary. Your regular physician has the advantage of being someone you already know and trust, so you may feel most comfortable with this option.

For unimproved joint pain.   If you're experiencing pain that has not improved after a reasonable time—say, two weeks—you should consult with a rheumatologist. This is true even if you're already seeing a medical doctor for your condition. Rheumatologists have far more experience than do internists or family practitioners in recognizing the symptoms of diseases that affect the joints.

Finding a Good Arthritis Doctor

If you need to see a rheumatologist, that is, an arthritis doctor, you'll want to find one who has been certified by the American Board of Rheumatology. A certified rheumatologist has completed an approved residency program and passed a rigorous written exam in internal medicine, administered by the board, and has completed an approved fellowship training program in rheumatology. The fellowship program usually consists of two or three years of very specialized arthritis training. Once this training is complete, the doctor must then also pass a written test in rheumatology. All of this is a way of ensuring that your doctor knows what she/he is doing. This is especially important because any physician who graduates from medical school can legally claim to be a specialist, even without any specific training in the specialty. Here is how to start your search:

Ask your medical physician for a rheumatology referral.   Your family physician may refer you to an orthopedist, but don't agree to go unless you're interested in surgery. See a rheumatologist. If you had a heart problem, your doctor would have you see a cardiologist, not a heart surgeon. If you had colitis, you physician would have you see a gastroenterologist, not a colon surgeon. The same should be true for your arthritis, even if only to obtain a second opinion. If a medical doctor discourages you from seeking a second opinion, see it as a red warning flag and consider going elsewhere for your general medical needs and referrals.

Contact your local county Arthritis Foundation.   The Arthritis Foundation has a lot of wonderful information for patients or families of patients with arthritis. They also have a list of Board-Certified Rheumatologists in your area. You can find their national website at: www.arthritis.org.

Contact the American College of Rheumatology (ACR).   This is an organization that supports education, research, advocacy, and practice support programs for professionals in rheumatology. You can reach them at:

American College of Rheumatology
1800 Century Place, Suite 250
Atlanta, GA 30345–4300
Phone: 404 633 3777
www.rheumatology.org

The ACR's website, which is available to everyone, doctors and lay people alike, offers a list of all its members, both nationally and internationally. One caveat: doctors aren't required to have board certification to become members of the ACR, so you will need to ask about it if you contact a physician listed on the site. By the way, I would advise you to ask specifically if the doctor you're considering is board certified in rheumatology. I have seen physicians who have only certification in internal medicine say that they are indeed board certified, leaving out the fact that their certification is in internal medicine, not rheumatology.

MAKING LIFE A LITTLE EASIER

A small bag of frozen peas makes a great ice pack for sore or swollen joints. Just wrap the bag of peas in a towel and place it over the joint. The bag will mold to the shape of the joint.

Contact your local county or your state medical board, society, or association. Often, you can find websites for these organizations online. Do a web search that includes your state's name and the word medical. The appropriate organization will generally appear somewhere on the first page of listings.

Contact the medical staff office of your local hospital. Hospitals and clinics are often more than happy to direct people to appropriate physicians who practice in the local area.

Contact the staff office or Department of Medicine in a local medical school. Most medical schools and teaching hospitals will have highly-qualified rheumatologists on staff.

What to Expect

You have a right and duty to your own health to expect an adequate standard of care from any doctor you see. If you're being examined for joint problems, here's what you should absolutely look for:

A detailed history should be taken of your joint pain.   The characteristics of your discomfort can be of great help in diagnosing your condition. At a minimum, you should be asked the following questions:

- When did the pain begin?
- What joints are involved?
- What is the character of the pain? Is it sharp? Is it dull?
- Does the pain radiate (start at one point and go to another)?
- Is the pain constant or intermittent?
- Does the pain have varying degrees of intensity?
- What makes the pain worse? What makes the pain better?
- On a scale of 0 to 10 (0 being no pain, 10 being the worst pain), where is your pain?
- Is the pain worse in the morning when you wake up, or is it worse as the day goes on?
- Do you have any other body symptoms, such as fevers, rash, headache, muscle pain, or cough?

You should receive a detailed physical examination.   Of course your doctor should examine the joint or joints that hurt, but he/she should also look at all of your other joints. Although you may have pain in one joint, it would not be uncommon to have problems that you are not aware of in other joints. Knowing whether a problem is localized or involves many joints is very important in helping to make a diagnosis. If your knee hurts, for example, do not accept an evaluation that is based solely on examining that knee. If your doctor doesn't do more, thank him/her, limp out of the office, and make a beeline to your nearest rheumatologist. In addition to examining all of your joints, she/he should also look in your mouth for sores, listen to your lungs and heart, and feel your belly to make certain that there is no abdominal tenderness. Finally—and I can't stress this enough—you should receive a neurological exam. Many nerve problems present as joint pain, which is something that many doctors overlook.

You should have x-ray studies.   Do not accept any diagnosis of arthritis without having an x-ray to substantiate it. I can't tell you how many times I have seen patients who have been told, with no corroborating evidence, they have arthritis. You can't make a diagnosis without all of the available facts, and that includes an x-ray.

You should have laboratory tests.   Blood and urine tests can give us a great deal of information. Since *many illnesses* may present with joint pain, it is important to make certain that these illnesses are excluded. I usually obtain routine blood chemistries, a complete blood count (CBC), and a urinalysis. You should also have some specialized tests, including an immune system study called a *rheumatoid factor*, a test for lupus called an *anti-nuclear antibody* (ANA) test, and a test for inflammation called an *erythrocyte sedimentation rate* (ESR). Two newer tests are also important. This includes a very specific test for RA called a *cyclic citrullinated peptide* (CCP) antibody and a sensitive test for inflammation called a *C-reactive protein* (CRP).

You may be referred to an *occupational therapist* or a *physical therapist*. Although occupational and physical therapy are often mentioned in the same breath and are complementary to each other—both can play a vital role in helping you cope with your arthritis—they are also very different.

Physical therapy (PT) uses exercise to restore strength, endurance, and range of motion to a joint. In the case of arthritis, the goal is to help you regain greater use of joints that have become stiff and immobile from swelling and pain.

Whenever I recommend that a patient see a physical therapist, it's not uncommon for him or her to say, "I get plenty of exercise on my own. I belong to a health club." But it's important to realize that PT movements, under the supervision of a therapist, are more targeted and precise than those you do at the gym. Not only can they can help reduce the discomfort in your joints, but they can also teach you how to move *without doing any further damage.* In addition to exercise, your PT therapist may use other treatment options as well, including:

- Hot packs to increase blood flow to a specific site in the body.
- Cold packs to reduce swelling and inflammation.
- Water therapy, including exercising in a pool or spending time in a whirlpool.
- Massage to relax muscles and improve circulation.
- Transcutaneous (or galvanic) electrical nerve stimulation (TENS), which stimulates specific nerves with a very mild electrical current.
- Ultrasound, which uses high frequency sound waves to warm muscle fiber.
- Phonophoresis, which uses sound waves to help deliver medication through the skin.
- Iontophoresis, which uses a mild electrical current to help deliver medication through the skin.

The American Physical Therapy Association (APTA) is a national professional organization of physical therapists that fosters advancements in physical therapy practice, research, and education. You can learn more at the association's website: www.apta.org.

Occupational therapy (OT) trains you to move in a way that puts less strain on your joints and shows you how you can change your environment to help make performing the activities of daily living easier (see *Making Life a Little Easier* boxes throughout this book). Much of the training focuses on ways to move and use your shoulders, arms, wrists, hands, and fingers, and some of the treatments are the same as those used in PT. If your upper extremities are in a lot of pain, your therapist may give you a splint to wear.

The American Occupational Therapy Association (AOTA) is the nationally recognized professional association of occupational therapists, assistants, and students. You can learn more about occupational therapy at the association's website: www.aota.org.

MAKING LIFE A LITTLE EASIER

"Reachers and grabbers" are some of my patients' favorite aids. They allow you to pick up items from the floor or even help bring down objects from a shelf. These are great for patients who have difficulty bending down or reaching up. They are available in most hardware stores. Look for one that is lightweight and sturdy, and make sure you're comfortable with the handgrip. You don't have to use it only in the house. You can also take it to the store to help take items off the shelf and use it outside to pick up objects on the ground such as a ball or a toy.

A Word About the Internet

The World Wide Web is one of the best places to find general information about many subjects, but it is one of the worst sources of medical information. There are many good sites on the Web for patients, but there are also many sites that are less than reputable. Many of these sites have hidden agendas and want to sell you something. They often portray rheumatologic illness in the worst possible way in an attempt to scare you. You have no way to put the information into proper perspective. If you use the Web, take in the information, but don't believe everything that you read. Use the information as a springboard for discussions with your doctor.

Working with your Doctor

The program in this book is designed to be both safe and effective in helping you keep your arthritic pain and inflammation under control. For mild to moderate arthritis, it may be all you need. If you need a doctor's help, however, it's important that he/she know about your diet, exercise, and supplements.

If you're an older adult, for example, he/she may want to adjust your caloric intake to make sure you're getting proper nutrition. He/she may want you to do your exercises, at least initially, under a physical therapist's supervision. Most importantly, he/she needs to know about any and all supplements you're taking—not just the ones mentioned in this book. Supplements put active chemicals in your body, and these chemicals can interact with prescription drugs to create unexpected side effects. Too much fish oil, for example, can heighten the blood-thinning effects of drugs like Coumadin, which can then cause bleeding from your internal blood vessels.

Your best bet for a good result when working with your doctor is to get from and give to him/her as much information as possible. With that kind of cooperative, team approach, you can almost certainly bring the pain, stiffness, and inflammation of your arthritis under control and enjoy the good life you deserve.

CHAPTER **11**

Medications

NO ONE LIKES taking medications, not even doctors and nurses. You run the risk of side effects; remembering to take your daily or weekly dose is annoying; and as we all know, prescriptions can take a big bite out of your budget. But if your arthritis has progressed to the point where diet, exercise, and supplements can't control your pain, swelling, and inflammation, adding medications to your program may be your only option. Note that I said, "add to" your program, not "substitute for." It's important that you continue following the routines you've established to control arthritis. The more effective strategies you use to attack the problem, the better your results are likely to be.

Also, remember that even with powerful medicines, we're still dealing with the art of the possible. There is no known remedy that will cure arthritis. We can, however, control the damage, and in the case of RA, reverse it if we catch the disease in its early stages.

Osteoarthritis

OA is the eventual breakdown of joint cartilage due to inflammation. At its advanced stage, it leaves you with bone rubbing against bone. Unfortunately, we don't know how to grow cartilage back. Our goal, then, is to slow or stop the progression of your OA and reduce your pain so that you can comfortably walk up steps, open doors, brush your hair, and perform all of the other activities of daily living.

OA medications fall into three categories:

- Oral analgesics
- Oral anti-inflammatories
- Injectable medications

Oral Analgesics

Tylenol (acetaminophen).   For many patients, simple analgesics such as Tylenol are more than adequate to control the pain of OA. However, you should know that this *not* an anti-inflammatory drug. Its only use is to kill pain. I don't recommend the arthritis strength version (800 mg) of these meds, especially for older adults (and obviously not for children). At high doses, acetaminophen can become very toxic to your liver, and it does tend to have a cumulative effect over time. As a safety precaution, I recommend that my patients take only 600 mg every six hours. It's safer. By the way, be sure to check the labels of any over-the-counter cold remedies you may be taking, as these may already contain acetaminophen. As a precaution, do *not* take any form of this drug if you've been drinking, if you drink heavily every day, or if you've been fasting.

Darvocet.   For those patients who don't have pain control with simple analgesics, we sometimes use medications containing mild narcotics such as Darvocet. This drug is a combination of acetaminophen and a mild codeine-like chemical (propoxyphene). The problem with Darvocet is that it is habit-forming, so you always run the risk of addiction with it. Be sure to discuss the benefits and risks with your doctor before you start taking a drug like this. Because it contains acetaminophen, all of the precautions that apply to Tylenol apply to this drug as well. Darvocet can also cause dizziness, especially if you take it in combination with antihistamines, alcohol, sedatives, antidepressants, or other pain relievers.

PRECAUTION

All of these drugs can be used safely and effectively in appropriate cases, and none of them should interfere with your 28-day program. Be sure to consult with your physician about the risks and benefits of whatever he/she recommends. A special note to pregnant women and women of childbearing years—many of these medications can be harmful to an unborn child. Several can cause birth defects, even if being used by a potential father when conception occurs.

Anti-inflammatories

Non-steroidal anti-inflammatory drugs (NSAIDs) have undergone some controversy lately because many of them have been shown to increase the risk of kidney problems, gastrointestinal bleeding, and heart disease. We certainly still use them, because they can be very effective, but you should take them only under a doctor's supervision—even the over-the-counter ones. Here are some of the more common ones:

Naprosyn, Anaprox (naproxen).   No one really knows how drugs like Naprosyn and other NSAIDs work, but they are very powerful painkillers. They have been used to treat not only OA, but RA, juvenile arthritis, and ankylosing spondylitis as well. As mentioned above, the problem with them is that they increase risk for heart attack, stroke, and very serious stomach ulcers. Don't take them if you already have circulatory or blood vessel disease.

Indocin (indomethacin).   This drug has the same potential adverse side effects as Naprosyn. Among the many conditions that should make you think twice about using this drug are a history of liver, kidney, stomach, bowel, or heart disease; diabetes; depression; Parkinson's disease, and many others. Again, discuss these issues with your doctor before deciding whether to use this drug.

Motrin (ibuprofen).   This is a very commonly used drug, but like other NSAIDs, its use poses significant risks to your health. All of the warnings that apply to Naprosyn and Indocin apply to this drug as well. Even though it is easily available over the counter, if you want to take it, do so only under a doctor's supervision.

Mobic (meloxicam).   Although this drug poses risks similar to other NSAIDs, the risks seem to be somewhat lower. Usually, the longer you use this drug, like any NSAID, the greater chance that you'll experience side effects. However, they can occur even after short-term use. Warning signs include:

- Black or tarry stools
- Dark urine
- Diarrhea
- Fatigue
- Generalized itching
- Indigestion, nausea, or vomiting
- Jaundice (yellow skin or eyes)
- Joint pain
- Nausea
- Stomach pain or burning
- Upper respiratory tract infection

Because the risks for heart, kidney, and stomach problems seem to be lower for meloxicam, it's the NSAID of choice for my patients.

MAKING LIFE A LITTLE EASIER

Pill splitters are an easy way to cut pills. They are inexpensive and allow you to save money when doses of your medications are changed. They are available at most drugstores.

Injectables

Not all medications are best taken by mouth. Some need to arrive directly at the inflamed joint itself. For that, you need an injectable. There are two types:

- Corticosteroids
- Hyaluronic acid

Corticosteroids.   These drugs, which include *cortisone, prednisone, and methylprednisolone,* are powerful anti-inflammatory agents that are chemically similar to a stress hormone, cortisol, that the body produces naturally. By the way, even though we sometimes refer to these drugs simply as "steroids," they have nothing to do with the type of steroids athletes use to enhance their performance.

We really don't like to inject any one joint more than once every four months. Repeated injections can damage the joint, resulting in an increased risk for infection. Personally, if I have to inject somebody's joint more than twice a year, I get concerned that they may need to have that joint replaced surgically.

As a side note, before giving an injection of corticosteroids, we often aspirate any fluid that has accumulated around the inflammation. Fluid causes pressure on the inflamed joint, which then causes further cartilage damage. Of course, we can't do this for every joint. We can for the ankle, knee, shoulder, elbow, wrist, and hand, but there is really no way to do it for the hip.

Hyaluronic acid.   These are newer medicines, which have appeared in the last eight years or so. Brand names include Synvisc, Euflexxa, Orthovisc, Hyalgan, and Supartz. Hyaluronic acid is actually a type of carbohydrate, called an *aminoglycan,* that is a major component in the synovial fluid that protects your joints. We believe that it is largely responsible for the fluid's lubricating properties. The medications are not taken from human joints, of course, but from the combs of roosters, which are mostly composed of cartilage. When we inject the medicine into a joint, it incorporates into the cartilage at a microscopic level and helps protect and preserve it. The injections use a very thin needle and are virtually painless. Normally, you will be given one injection a week for anywhere from three to five weeks, depending on which product you're using. This medication works best in treating early disease. The further along the arthritis has developed, the less effective hyaluronic acid will be. The side effects are usually mild and local. They include pain, swelling, rash, and/or itching at the injection site.

Rheumatoid Arthritis

Unlike OA, RA is a disease that begins with the immune system. While we can use some of the same drugs to treat the pain and inflammation of both illnesses, we have some more powerful medications to attack the inflammation of RA. We try to start with the simplest ones, of course, and move toward the more potent drugs only if we have to.

Whatever we use, the most important consideration is that we treat RA early and aggressively. Studies show that if we do that, we can often bring RA inflammation under control. That is, we can slow down, prevent, or even reverse some of the damage that's been done to the joints.

In my own practice, I'll start an RA patient on an NSAID and see if I can bring the inflammation down in the joints in four to six weeks. If I can't, I will seriously start thinking about placing him/her on a *disease modifying anti-rheumatic drug* (DMARD). These are drugs for long-term treatment. Some are slow to take effect, and some are faster. But they all have the potential of putting the disease into remission or significantly slowing down its progression.

There is also a place for the use of corticosteroids. In somebody who has significant, acute inflammation, we may put them on an oral steroid taper of moderate to low dosage over a few weeks, just to get the joints under control. At that point, we may be able to get him/her on an NSAID or a DMARD.

Now there have been studies showing that those patients with RA who have been on a low dose, long-term course of Prednisone (less than 10 mg a day) have, over the years, suffered less damage to their joints than those patients who have not been on those drugs. However, they're double-edged swords. We would prefer not to have patients on them because of the potential risks of side effects. These side effects can include weight gain, mood swings, round face, hair loss or overgrowth, blurred vision, muscle loss and weakness, a swollen area on the back of the neck called a "buffalo hump," purple stretch marks, high blood pressure, high blood sugar, slow healing, bruising, and many more. To avoid these side effects, I will try a DMARD.

DMARDS

This class of drugs is used specifically with RA, and their advantage is that we can use them either to get patients off of corticosteroids or to avoid them altogether. Some are relatively mild, and some are potent enough to treat cancer.

Gold.   We used to use injectable gold quite a bit in treating RA. In fact, the medication has been around for seventy years. It was originally used to treat tuberculosis, and as it turned out, patients who had RA along with their tuberculosis saw their RA improve. There were several problems with gold. For one thing, it took about six months to work, and patients had to come in every week for an injection. Gold also had some serious side effects that made it undesirable, including kidney damage. You can still get injectable gold today, and there is an oral form on the market, but we now have better, more effective drugs for treating RA that I believe offer a better choice.

Plaquenil (hydroxychloroquine). This drug is a derivative of another, *chloroquine,* that was used to treat and prevent malaria among the American GIs in World War II. It turned out that GIs with RA who took the drug saw their arthritis get better. Chloroquine was highly toxic, but the hydroxyl form now in use proved much safer. In fact, it's considered one of our safest drugs. It's effective in about 50 to 60 percent of cases, and we often use it as a base drug, adding other drugs into it. In very rare cases, Plaquenil can cause toxicity in the eyes, so patients on the drug need to get their eyes checked every six months. Like gold, this medication can take up to six months to work.

Rheumatrex, Trexall (methotrexate). We have been using this drug for the past fifteen years. In high doses, it is used to treat cancer, but in lower doses, the FDA has approved its use in treating RA. We also use it to treat lupus and ankylosing spondylitis. It starts working in about four to six weeks and usually reaches its maximum effect in about three months. You can take it once a week in pill form, though sometimes we give it as an injection. It works for 80 to 90 percent of patients.

Many times we will use a combination of Plaquenil and methotrexate because the two work together and are very effective in combination. We may also start a patient on Prednisone, Plaquenil, and methotrexate together. The Prednisone will start working within a few days, the methotrexate will start working in about a month, and the Plaquenil will start working in about six months. So as the methotrexate works, we start lowering the Prednisone dose, and once the Plaquenil kicks in, we get them off the methotrexate.

Methotrexate can have many side effects and if misused, can be extremely toxic. People who have accidentally taken their pill once a day rather than once a week have died from toxicity. Your doctor will probably want to do blood tests on a regular basis to check your kidney and liver function if you're taking this drug.

MAKING LIFE A LITTLE EASIER

If you are on multiple medications, a seven-day pillbox is wonderful. Each day is divided into morning, lunch, afternoon, and evening compartments. These are available at most drugstores.

Biologics.   The biologics are basically genetically engineered, designer medicines. These are the newest medications we use, and they work by inhibiting the immune system's production of certain substances that fuel the fire of RA inflammation. One of these substances is called *tumor necrosis factor* (TNF) and the other is *interleukin–1.*

There are three anti-TNF medications on the market: Enbrel (etanercept), Humira (adalimumab), and Remicade (infliximab). Humira and Enbrel are given by injection. Humira is given once every other week, while Enbrel is given every week. Remicade is given through an intravenous infusion once every two months. With all of these drugs, the main side effect is a tendency to develop infections, but this is usually easy to manage.

Kineret (anakinra) is a similar drug but inhibits interleukin–1 instead of TNF. The side effects are much the same as those for the anti-TNF medications.

Lesser Medications

There are a number of other medications that we use less frequently, either because they're not as effective as those mentioned above or because of potential side effects. Here are some of them:

Minocycline.   This is an antibiotic, and it's effective in about 40 percent of patients for mild disease. One of the problems with minocycline is that it causes skin discoloration in a fair number of patients, and that's enough to cause many to stop using the drug.

Imuran (azathioprine).   This drug is also approved by the FDA to treat RA, but it has significant side effects. It's an immunosuppressive agent that can reduce the number of blood cells in your bone marrow, and it increases your risk for skin cancer and lymphoma. It works in about 50 percent of patients.

Orencia (abatacept).   This is an artificially-made protein that keeps your immune system's T-cells from attacking the healthy tissue in joints. It's given through a monthly infusion into your veins. If you have or have ever had any serious lung disease, such as chronic obstructive pulmonary disease or tuberculosis, you may not be able to use Orencia, which can make breathing problems worse.

Rituxan (rituximab).   This works by selectively depleting certain B-cells from the immune system. It's also used against non-Hodgkin's lymphoma, a deadly form of lymphatic cancer. Side effects are rare, but can include fever and chills. Both Orencia and Rituxan are used to treat patients with more advanced disease. Like Orencia, Rituxan is given through an intravenous infusion.

Arava (leflunomide).   This is also an immunosuppressive agent given orally. It's effective in 80 to 90 percent of patients. We really can't give it to women in their childbearing years. Although rare, Arava has caused liver injury and death to some patients. It has also caused interstitial lung disease, a dangerous inflammation of lung lining.

Azulfidine (sulfasalazine).   This is an oral drug that is effective in about half of all patients but it can take three to six months to work. Side effects can include aches, rashes, diarrhea, dizziness, headache, light sensitivity, itching, appetite loss, liver problems, lowered blood count, nausea, or vomiting.

APPENDIX A:
WEEKLY MEAL PLAN NUTRITION CHARTS

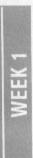

DAY 1

Breakfast

Amount Per Serving	
Calories	349.90
Calories From Fat (13%)	45.58
	% Daily Value
Total Fat 5.51g	**8%**
Saturated Fat 0.45g	**2%**
Cholesterol 0.00mg	**0%**
Sodium 473.45mg	**20%**
Potassium 828.45mg	**24%**
Carbohydrates 70.72g	**24%**
Dietary Fiber 10.07g	**40%**
Sugar 8.58g	
Sugar Alcohols 0.00g	
Net Carbohydrates 60.65g	
Protein 9.99g	**20%**

Lunch

Amount Per Serving	
Calories	365.61
Calories From Fat (16%)	57.84
	% Daily Value
Total Fat 6.57g	**10%**
Saturated Fat 1.18g	**6%**
Cholesterol 36.12mg	**12%**
Sodium 305.48mg	**13%**
Potassium 954.88mg	**27%**
Carbohydrates 52.56g	**18%**
Dietary Fiber 11.19g	**45%**
Sugar 10.29g	
Sugar Alcohols 0.00g	
Net Carbohydrates 41.37g	
Protein 26.68g	**53%**

Dinner

Amount Per Serving	
Calories	739.32
Calories From Fat (47%)	344.84
	% Daily Value
Total Fat 40.58g	**62%**
Saturated Fat 5.35g	**27%**
Cholesterol 68.44mg	**23%**
Sodium 395.78mg	**16%**
Potassium 1759.49mg	**50%**
Carbohydrates 58.59g	**20%**
Dietary Fiber 15.86g	**63%**
Sugar 7.66g	
Sugar Alcohols 0.00g	
Net Carbohydrates 42.73g	
Protein 44.51g	**89%**

Evening Snack

Amount Per Serving	
Calories	115.99
Calories From Fat (1%)	1.66
	% Daily Value
Total Fat 0.20g	**0%**
Saturated Fat 0.01g	**0%**
Cholesterol 7.00mg	**2%**
Sodium 70.31mg	**3%**
Potassium 266.43mg	**8%**
Carbohydrates 24.67g	**8%**
Dietary Fiber 2.00g	**8%**
Sugar 20.36g	
Sugar Alcohols 0.00g	
Net Carbohydrates 22.67g	
Protein 4.37g	**9%**

See p. 122 for complete meal.

DAY 2

Breakfast

Amount Per Serving		
Calories	592.14	
Calories From Fat (32%)	191.48	
		% Daily Value
Total Fat 22.23g		**34%**
Saturated Fat 2.12g		**11%**
Cholesterol 2.45mg		**1%**
Sodium 234.53mg		**10%**
Potassium 1003.04mg		**29%**
Carbohydrates 93.21g		**31%**
Dietary Fiber 10.49g		**42%**
Sugar 55.70g		
Sugar Alcohols 0.00g		
Net Carbohydrates 82.71g		
Protein 13.33g		**27%**

Lunch

Amount Per Serving		
Calories	525.35	
Calories From Fat (27%)	139.63	
		% Daily Value
Total Fat 16.37g		**25%**
Saturated Fat 2.04g		**10%**
Cholesterol 34.22mg		**11%**
Sodium 302.31mg		**13%**
Potassium 1123.50mg		**32%**
Carbohydrates 81.22g		**27%**
Dietary Fiber 11.67g		**47%**
Sugar 42.52g		
Sugar Alcohols 0.00g		
Net Carbohydrates 69.54g		
Protein 22.68g		**45%**

Dinner

Amount Per Serving		
Calories	336.24	
Calories From Fat (23%)	78.29	
		% Daily Value
Total Fat 8.85g		**14%**
Saturated Fat 1.27g		**6%**
Cholesterol 46.75mg		**16%**
Sodium 429.44mg		**18%**
Potassium 888.52mg		**25%**
Carbohydrates 41.63g		**14%**
Dietary Fiber 6.66g		**27%**
Sugar 11.15g		
Sugar Alcohols 0.00g		
Net Carbohydrates 34.97g		
Protein 23.39g		**47%**

Evening Snack

Amount Per Serving		
Calories	127.28	
Calories From Fat (65%)	82.71	
		% Daily Value
Total Fat 8.66g		**13%**
Saturated Fat 5.01g		**25%**
Cholesterol 1.00mg		**0%**
Sodium 10.54mg		**0%**
Potassium 82.62mg		**2%**
Carbohydrates 10.65g		**4%**
Dietary Fiber 2.08g		**8%**
Sugar 8.14g		
Sugar Alcohols 0.00g		
Net Carbohydrates 8.57g		
Protein 0.36g		**1%**

See p. 123 for complete meal.

DAY 3

Breakfast

Amount Per Serving		
Calories		286.57
Calories From Fat (11%)		31.63
		% Daily Value
Total Fat 3.60g		**6%**
Saturated Fat 0.64g		**3%**
Cholesterol 0.63mg		**0%**
Sodium 170.18mg		**7%**
Potassium 806.63mg		**23%**
Carbohydrates 53.90g		**18%**
Dietary Fiber 1.98g		**8%**
Sugar 35.31g		
Sugar Alcohols 0.00g		
Net Carbohydrates 51.92g		
Protein 11.61g		**23%**

Lunch

Amount Per Serving		
Calories		313.70
Calories From Fat (45%)		139.76
		% Daily Value
Total Fat 16.16g		**25%**
Saturated Fat 4.50g		**23%**
Cholesterol 22.25mg		**7%**
Sodium 932.12mg		**39%**
Potassium 904.76mg		**26%**
Carbohydrates 34.13g		**11%**
Dietary Fiber 8.87g		**35%**
Sugar 8.89g		
Sugar Alcohols 0.00g		
Net Carbohydrates 25.25g		
Protein 11.77g		**24%**

Dinner

Amount Per Serving		
Calories		696.37
Calories From Fat (23%)		161.45
		% Daily Value
Total Fat 18.51g		**28%**
Saturated Fat 2.27g		**11%**
Cholesterol 111.25mg		**37%**
Sodium 574.20mg		**24%**
Potassium 4145.49mg		**118%**
Carbohydrates 95.08g		**32%**
Dietary Fiber 20.46g		**82%**
Sugar 55.24g		
Sugar Alcohols 0.00g		
Net Carbohydrates 74.62g		
Protein 48.77g		**98%**

Evening Snack

Amount Per Serving		
Calories		238.13
Calories From Fat (59%)		141.39
		% Daily Value
Total Fat 16.09g		**25%**
Saturated Fat 10.21g		**51%**
Cholesterol 62.73mg		**21%**
Sodium 103.78mg		**4%**
Potassium 159.19mg		**5%**
Carbohydrates 9.23g		**3%**
Dietary Fiber 0.89g		**4%**
Sugar 4.15g		
Sugar Alcohols 0.00g		
Net Carbohydrates 8.35g		
Protein 14.12g		**28%**

See p. 124 for complete meal.

DAY 4

Breakfast

Amount Per Serving		
Calories		496.28
Calories From Fat (16%)		81.80
		% Daily Value
Total Fat 9.54g		**15%**
Saturated Fat 2.92g		**15%**
Cholesterol 14.94mg		**5%**
Sodium 186.16mg		**8%**
Potassium 777.08mg		**22%**
Carbohydrates 87.47g		**29%**
Dietary Fiber 9.81g		**39%**
Sugar 7.80g		
Sugar Alcohols 0.00g		
Net Carbohydrates 77.65g		
Protein 21.39g		**43%**

Lunch

Amount Per Serving		
Calories		471.00
Calories From Fat (40%)		188.25
		% Daily Value
Total Fat 22.17g		**34%**
Saturated Fat 2.75g		**14%**
Cholesterol 0.00mg		**0%**
Sodium 416.90mg		**17%**
Potassium 1275.97mg		**36%**
Carbohydrates 58.71g		**20%**
Dietary Fiber 20.16g		**81%**
Sugar 3.60g		
Sugar Alcohols 0.00g		
Net Carbohydrates 38.54g		
Protein 16.67g		**33%**

Dinner

Amount Per Serving		
Calories		473.31
Calories From Fat (42%)		198.76
		% Daily Value
Total Fat 22.59g		**35%**
Saturated Fat 2.64g		**13%**
Cholesterol 207.19mg		**69%**
Sodium 572.73mg		**24%**
Potassium 1117.45mg		**32%**
Carbohydrates 35.10g		**12%**
Dietary Fiber 7.15g		**29%**
Sugar 8.50g		
Sugar Alcohols 0.00g		
Net Carbohydrates 27.96g		
Protein 29.62g		**59%**

Evening Snack

Amount Per Serving		
Calories		83.41
Calories From Fat (5%)		4.49
		% Daily Value
Total Fat 0.54g		**1%**
Saturated Fat 0.03g		**0%**
Cholesterol 0.00mg		**0%**
Sodium 0.37mg		**0%**
Potassium 319.81mg		**9%**
Carbohydrates 20.20g		**7%**
Dietary Fiber 3.91g		**16%**
Sugar 16.53g		
Sugar Alcohols 0.00g		
Net Carbohydrates 16.30g		
Protein 1.78g		**4%**

WEEK 1

See p. 125 for complete meal.

DAY 5

Breakfast

Amount Per Serving		
Calories	439.35	
Calories From Fat (40%)	175.37	
		% Daily Value
Total Fat 19.85g		**31%**
Saturated Fat 2.85g		**14%**
Cholesterol 4.30mg		**1%**
Sodium 400.36mg		**17%**
Potassium 1015.19mg		**29%**
Carbohydrates 44.69g		**15%**
Dietary Fiber 6.00g		**24%**
Sugar 21.83g		
Sugar Alcohols 0.00g		
Net Carbohydrates 38.69g		
Protein 22.95g		**46%**

Lunch

Amount Per Serving		
Calories	220.92	
Calories From Fat (57%)	125.18	
		% Daily Value
Total Fat 14.26g		**22%**
Saturated Fat 1.38g		**7%**
Cholesterol 0.00mg		**0%**
Sodium 183.37mg		**8%**
Potassium 931.89mg		**27%**
Carbohydrates 21.97g		**7%**
Dietary Fiber 4.97g		**20%**
Sugar 13.83g		
Sugar Alcohols 0.00g		
Net Carbohydrates 17.00g		
Protein 3.62g		**7%**

Dinner

Amount Per Serving		
Calories	514.28	
Calories From Fat (49%)	253.00	
		% Daily Value
Total Fat 29.63g		**46%**
Saturated Fat 3.72g		**19%**
Cholesterol 38.25mg		**13%**
Sodium 590.14mg		**25%**
Potassium 1293.49mg		**37%**
Carbohydrates 42.50g		**14%**
Dietary Fiber 5.69g		**23%**
Sugar 13.27g		
Sugar Alcohols 0.00g		
Net Carbohydrates 36.81g		
Protein 25.98g		**52%**

Evening Snack

Amount Per Serving		
Calories	127.28	
Calories From Fat (65%)	82.71	
		% Daily Value
Total Fat 8.66g		**13%**
Saturated Fat 5.01g		**25%**
Cholesterol 1.00mg		**0%**
Sodium 10.54mg		**0%**
Potassium 82.62mg		**2%**
Carbohydrates 10.65g		**4%**
Dietary Fiber 2.08g		**8%**
Sugar 8.14g		
Sugar Alcohols 0.00g		
Net Carbohydrates 8.57g		
Protein 0.36g		**1%**

See p. 126 for complete meal.

DAY 6

Breakfast

Amount Per Serving		
Calories	322.32	
Calories From Fat (23%)	75.50	
		% Daily Value
Total Fat 8.86g		**14%**
Saturated Fat 2.06g		**10%**
Cholesterol 9.74mg		**3%**
Sodium 663.23mg		**28%**
Potassium 602.66mg		**17%**
Carbohydrates 45.41g		**15%**
Dietary Fiber 8.20g		**33%**
Sugar 9.30g		
Sugar Alcohols 0.00g		
Net Carbohydrates 37.21g		
Protein 19.10g		**38%**

Lunch

Amount Per Serving		
Calories	462.98	
Calories From Fat (28%)	129.30	
		% Daily Value
Total Fat 15.11g		**23%**
Saturated Fat 2.33g		**12%**
Cholesterol 0.00mg		**0%**
Sodium 294.74mg		**12%**
Potassium 1286.29mg		**37%**
Carbohydrates 76.24g		**25%**
Dietary Fiber 12.13g		**49%**
Sugar 39.11g		
Sugar Alcohols 0.00g		
Net Carbohydrates 64.10g		
Protein 11.89g		**24%**

Dinner

Amount Per Serving		
Calories	549.39	
Calories From Fat (25%)	136.04	
		% Daily Value
Total Fat 15.27g		**23%**
Saturated Fat 5.69g		**28%**
Cholesterol 55.23mg		**18%**
Sodium 1224.20mg		**51%**
Potassium 1367.98mg		**39%**
Carbohydrates 61.47g		**20%**
Dietary Fiber 35.35g		**141%**
Sugar 6.57g		
Sugar Alcohols 0.00g		
Net Carbohydrates 26.12g		
Protein 43.81g		**88%**

Evening Snack

Amount Per Serving		
Calories	210.04	
Calories From Fat (45%)	94.47	
		% Daily Value
Total Fat 10.84g		**17%**
Saturated Fat 3.97g		**20%**
Cholesterol 5.50mg		**2%**
Sodium 60.46mg		**3%**
Potassium 79.51mg		**2%**
Carbohydrates 26.95g		**9%**
Dietary Fiber 6.00g		**24%**
Sugar 18.30g		
Sugar Alcohols 0.00g		
Net Carbohydrates 20.95g		
Protein 4.51g		**9%**

See p. 127 for complete meal.

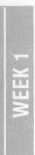

WEEK 1

DAY 7

Breakfast

Amount Per Serving		
Calories	359.93	
Calories From Fat (21%)	74.18	
		% Daily Value
Total Fat 8.96g		**14%**
Saturated Fat 0.99g		**5%**
Cholesterol 2.45mg		**1%**
Sodium 319.50mg		**13%**
Potassium 784.55mg		**22%**
Carbohydrates 65.73g		**22%**
Dietary Fiber 8.38g		**34%**
Sugar 30.82g		
Sugar Alcohols 0.00g		
Net Carbohydrates 57.35g		
Protein 10.94g		**22%**

Lunch

Amount Per Serving		
Calories	407.66	
Calories From Fat (29%)	118.92	
		% Daily Value
Total Fat 13.22g		**20%**
Saturated Fat 5.82g		**29%**
Cholesterol 56.02mg		**19%**
Sodium 529.51mg		**22%**
Potassium 808.00mg		**23%**
Carbohydrates 36.08g		**12%**
Dietary Fiber 4.95g		**20%**
Sugar 4.01g		
Sugar Alcohols 0.00g		
Net Carbohydrates 31.13g		
Protein 37.48g		**75%**

Dinner

Amount Per Serving		
Calories	724.99	
Calories From Fat (41%)	296.62	
		% Daily Value
Total Fat 34.21g		**53%**
Saturated Fat 3.46g		**17%**
Cholesterol 39.95mg		**13%**
Sodium 1161.25mg		**48%**
Potassium 1415.88mg		**40%**
Carbohydrates 60.49g		**20%**
Dietary Fiber 12.48g		**50%**
Sugar 16.21g		
Sugar Alcohols 0.00g		
Net Carbohydrates 48.00g		
Protein 32.17g		**64%**

Evening Snack

Amount Per Serving		
Calories	49.56	
Calories From Fat (11%)	5.40	
		% Daily Value
Total Fat 0.64g		**1%**
Saturated Fat 0.19g		**1%**
Cholesterol 1.02mg		**0%**
Sodium 14.30mg		**1%**
Potassium 163.43mg		**5%**
Carbohydrates 10.07g		**3%**
Dietary Fiber 4.03g		**16%**
Sugar 6.35g		
Sugar Alcohols 0.00g		
Net Carbohydrates 6.03g		
Protein 2.02g		**4%**

See p. 128 for complete meal.

DAY 8

Breakfast

Amount Per Serving		
Calories	196.14	
Calories From Fat (22%)	43.93	
		% Daily Value
Total Fat 4.98g		8%
Saturated Fat 0.48g		2%
Cholesterol 0.00mg		0%
Sodium 986.57mg		41%
Potassium 1080.53mg		31%
Carbohydrates 20.54g		7%
Dietary Fiber 3.82g		15%
Sugar 12.29g		
Sugar Alcohols 0.00g		
Net Carbohydrates 16.72g		
Protein 17.69g		35%

Lunch

Amount Per Serving		
Calories	384.48	
Calories From Fat (43%)	166.14	
		% Daily Value
Total Fat 19.09g		29%
Saturated Fat 2.44g		12%
Cholesterol 14.84mg		5%
Sodium 494.45mg		21%
Potassium 677.23mg		19%
Carbohydrates 28.39g		9%
Dietary Fiber 6.80g		27%
Sugar 6.00g		
Sugar Alcohols 0.00g		
Net Carbohydrates 21.60g		
Protein 28.09g		56%

Dinner

Amount Per Serving		
Calories	607.83	
Calories From Fat (23%)	139.36	
		% Daily Value
Total Fat 16.08g		25%
Saturated Fat 1.85g		9%
Cholesterol 0.00mg		0%
Sodium 446.20mg		19%
Potassium 1613.12mg		46%
Carbohydrates 103.87g		35%
Dietary Fiber 17.55g		70%
Sugar 15.37g		
Sugar Alcohols 0.00g		
Net Carbohydrates 86.32g		
Protein 17.45g		35%

Evening Snack

Amount Per Serving		
Calories	210.04	
Calories From Fat (45%)	94.47	
		% Daily Value
Total Fat 10.84g		17%
Saturated Fat 3.97g		20%
Cholesterol 5.50mg		2%
Sodium 60.46mg		3%
Potassium 79.51mg		2%
Carbohydrates 26.95g		9%
Dietary Fiber 6.00g		24%
Sugar 18.30g		
Sugar Alcohols 0.00g		
Net Carbohydrates 20.95g		
Protein 4.51g		9%

WEEK 2

See p. 129 for complete meal.

DAY 9

WEEK 2

Breakfast

Amount Per Serving		
Calories	449.18	
Calories From Fat (15%)	69.48	
		% Daily Value
Total Fat 8.44g		**13%**
Saturated Fat 0.83g		**4%**
Cholesterol 2.45mg		**1%**
Sodium 72.43mg		**3%**
Potassium 691.48mg		**20%**
Carbohydrates 89.69g		**30%**
Dietary Fiber 9.63g		**39%**
Sugar 51.32g		
Sugar Alcohols 0.00g		
Net Carbohydrates 80.06g		
Protein 12.57g		**25%**

Lunch

Amount Per Serving		
Calories	522.13	
Calories From Fat (49%)	257.54	
		% Daily Value
Total Fat 29.89g		**46%**
Saturated Fat 3.96g		**20%**
Cholesterol 172.37mg		**57%**
Sodium 182.48mg		**8%**
Potassium 914.46mg		**26%**
Carbohydrates 39.86g		**13%**
Dietary Fiber 9.81g		**39%**
Sugar 15.59g		
Sugar Alcohols 0.00g		
Net Carbohydrates 30.04g		
Protein 27.92g		**56%**

Dinner

Amount Per Serving		
Calories	562.14	
Calories From Fat (23%)	131.38	
		% Daily Value
Total Fat 14.95g		**23%**
Saturated Fat 1.93g		**10%**
Cholesterol 44.07mg		**15%**
Sodium 1089.82mg		**45%**
Potassium 2524.17mg		**72%**
Carbohydrates 85.65g		**29%**
Dietary Fiber 5.08g		**20%**
Sugar 5.36g		
Sugar Alcohols 0.00g		
Net Carbohydrates 80.57g		
Protein 27.93g		**56%**

Evening Snack

Amount Per Serving		
Calories	83.41	
Calories From Fat (5%)	4.49	
		% Daily Value
Total Fat 0.54g		**1%**
Saturated Fat 0.03g		**0%**
Cholesterol 0.00mg		**0%**
Sodium 0.37mg		**0%**
Potassium 319.81mg		**9%**
Carbohydrates 20.20g		**7%**
Dietary Fiber 3.91g		**16%**
Sugar 16.53g		
Sugar Alcohols 0.00g		
Net Carbohydrates 16.30g		
Protein 1.78g		**4%**

See p. 130 for complete meal.

DAY 10

Breakfast

Amount Per Serving	
Calories	399.20
Calories From Fat (23%)	91.47
	% Daily Value
Total Fat 10.59g	**16%**
Saturated Fat 2.48g	**12%**
Cholesterol 22.78mg	**8%**
Sodium 1664.10mg	**69%**
Potassium 628.35mg	**18%**
Carbohydrates 48.89g	**16%**
Dietary Fiber 5.80g	**23%**
Sugar 4.87g	
Sugar Alcohols 0.00g	
Net Carbohydrates 43.09g	
Protein 29.71g	**59%**

Lunch

Amount Per Serving	
Calories	231.42
Calories From Fat (41%)	94.51
	% Daily Value
Total Fat 11.04g	**17%**
Saturated Fat 1.19g	**6%**
Cholesterol 18.81mg	**6%**
Sodium 254.88mg	**11%**
Potassium 572.51mg	**16%**
Carbohydrates 23.06g	**8%**
Dietary Fiber 5.93g	**24%**
Sugar 2.32g	
Sugar Alcohols 0.00g	
Net Carbohydrates 17.13g	
Protein 13.40g	**27%**

Dinner

Amount Per Serving	
Calories	601.52
Calories From Fat (18%)	110.48
	% Daily Value
Total Fat 12.60g	**19%**
Saturated Fat 1.86g	**9%**
Cholesterol 46.75mg	**16%**
Sodium 828.75mg	**35%**
Potassium 1268.71mg	**36%**
Carbohydrates 88.74g	**30%**
Dietary Fiber 39.71g	**159%**
Sugar 12.21g	
Sugar Alcohols 0.00g	
Net Carbohydrates 49.03g	
Protein 33.18g	**66%**

Evening Snack

Amount Per Serving	
Calories	210.04
Calories From Fat (45%)	94.47
	% Daily Value
Total Fat 10.84g	**17%**
Saturated Fat 3.97g	**20%**
Cholesterol 5.50mg	**2%**
Sodium 60.46mg	**3%**
Potassium 79.51mg	**2%**
Carbohydrates 26.95g	**9%**
Dietary Fiber 6.00g	**24%**
Sugar 18.30g	
Sugar Alcohols 0.00g	
Net Carbohydrates 20.95g	
Protein 4.51g	**9%**

WEEK 2

See p. 131 for complete meal.

DAY 11

Breakfast

Amount Per Serving		
Calories	588.23	
Calories From Fat (40%)	234.40	
		% Daily Value
Total Fat 27.57g		42%
Saturated Fat 3.44g		17%
Cholesterol 9.15mg		3%
Sodium 151.12mg		6%
Potassium 810.83mg		23%
Carbohydrates 77.67g		26%
Dietary Fiber 9.71g		39%
Sugar 27.26g		
Sugar Alcohols 0.00g		
Net Carbohydrates 67.96g		
Protein 14.83g		30%

Lunch

Amount Per Serving		
Calories	481.02	
Calories From Fat (25%)	122.03	
		% Daily Value
Total Fat 14.29g		22%
Saturated Fat 3.55g		18%
Cholesterol 14.94mg		5%
Sodium 178.77mg		7%
Potassium 1350.75mg		39%
Carbohydrates 78.55g		26%
Dietary Fiber 8.85g		35%
Sugar 41.05g		
Sugar Alcohols 0.00g		
Net Carbohydrates 69.70g		
Protein 17.85g		36%

Dinner

Amount Per Serving		
Calories	390.68	
Calories From Fat (19%)	76.01	
		% Daily Value
Total Fat 8.67g		13%
Saturated Fat 1.13g		6%
Cholesterol 38.25mg		13%
Sodium 868.12mg		36%
Potassium 971.21mg		28%
Carbohydrates 56.22g		19%
Dietary Fiber 8.82g		35%
Sugar 21.53g		
Sugar Alcohols 0.00g		
Net Carbohydrates 47.39g		
Protein 25.73g		51%

Evening Snack

Amount Per Serving		
Calories	49.56	
Calories From Fat (11%)	5.40	
		% Daily Value
Total Fat 0.64g		1%
Saturated Fat 0.19g		1%
Cholesterol 1.02mg		0%
Sodium 14.30mg		1%
Potassium 163.43mg		5%
Carbohydrates 10.07g		3%
Dietary Fiber 4.03g		16%
Sugar 6.35g		
Sugar Alcohols 0.00g		
Net Carbohydrates 6.03g		
Protein 2.02g		4%

See p. 132 for complete meal.

DAY 12

Breakfast

Amount Per Serving		
Calories	640.20	
Calories From Fat (17%)	105.84	
		% Daily Value
Total Fat 12.58g		19%
Saturated Fat 2.03g		10%
Cholesterol 7.47mg		2%
Sodium 140.05mg		6%
Potassium 835.81mg		24%
Carbohydrates 120.58g		40%
Dietary Fiber 11.82g		47%
Sugar 36.40g		
Sugar Alcohols 0.00g		
Net Carbohydrates 108.76g		
Protein 19.15g		38%

Lunch

Amount Per Serving		
Calories	374.28	
Calories From Fat (62%)	233.11	
		% Daily Value
Total Fat 27.47g		42%
Saturated Fat 4.48g		22%
Cholesterol 0.00mg		0%
Sodium 125.98mg		5%
Potassium 1133.96mg		32%
Carbohydrates 28.37g		9%
Dietary Fiber 11.17g		45%
Sugar 7.23g		
Sugar Alcohols 0.00g		
Net Carbohydrates 17.20g		
Protein 11.43g		23%

Dinner

Amount Per Serving		
Calories	482.11	
Calories From Fat (27%)	128.35	
		% Daily Value
Total Fat 14.61g		22%
Saturated Fat 1.72g		9%
Cholesterol 68.44mg		23%
Sodium 662.09mg		28%
Potassium 1053.84mg		30%
Carbohydrates 54.98g		18%
Dietary Fiber 9.44g		38%
Sugar 18.37g		
Sugar Alcohols 0.00g		
Net Carbohydrates 45.53g		
Protein 35.47g		71%

WEEK 2

See p. 133 for complete meal.

DAY 13

Breakfast

Amount Per Serving	
Calories	433.46
Calories From Fat (43%)	184.77
	% Daily Value
Total Fat 20.95g	**32%**
Saturated Fat 2.81g	**14%**
Cholesterol 0.63mg	**0%**
Sodium 397.07mg	**17%**
Potassium 1282.45mg	**37%**
Carbohydrates 52.52g	**18%**
Dietary Fiber 3.87g	**15%**
Sugar 12.54g	
Sugar Alcohols 0.00g	
Net Carbohydrates 48.65g	
Protein 13.86g	**28%**

Lunch

Amount Per Serving	
Calories	467.83
Calories From Fat (27%)	126.54
	% Daily Value
Total Fat 14.94g	**23%**
Saturated Fat 1.62g	**8%**
Cholesterol 64.63mg	**22%**
Sodium 74.75mg	**3%**
Potassium 976.37mg	**28%**
Carbohydrates 76.15g	**25%**
Dietary Fiber 10.78g	**43%**
Sugar 42.29g	
Sugar Alcohols 0.00g	
Net Carbohydrates 65.37g	
Protein 15.92g	**32%**

Dinner

Amount Per Serving	
Calories	594.02
Calories From Fat (24%)	145.26
	% Daily Value
Total Fat 16.38g	**25%**
Saturated Fat 4.69g	**23%**
Cholesterol 151.30mg	**50%**
Sodium 896.54mg	**37%**
Potassium 1985.02mg	**57%**
Carbohydrates 52.13g	**17%**
Dietary Fiber 9.46g	**38%**
Sugar 17.26g	
Sugar Alcohols 0.00g	
Net Carbohydrates 42.66g	
Protein 60.29g	**121%**

Evening Snack

Amount Per Serving	
Calories	100.00
Calories From Fat (0%)	0.00
	% Daily Value
Total Fat 0.00g	**0%**
Saturated Fat 0.00g	**0%**
Cholesterol 7.00mg	**2%**
Sodium 70.00mg	**3%**
Potassium 220.00mg	**6%**
Carbohydrates 21.00g	**7%**
Dietary Fiber 0.00g	**0%**
Sugar 19.00g	
Sugar Alcohols 0.00g	
Net Carbohydrates 21.00g	
Protein 4.00g	**8%**

See p. 134 for complete meal.

WEEK 2

DAY 14

Breakfast

Amount Per Serving		
Calories	681.08	
Calories From Fat (33%)	221.77	
		% Daily Value
Total Fat 25.22g		39%
Saturated Fat 3.02g		15%
Cholesterol 2.78mg		1%
Sodium 830.32mg		35%
Potassium 922.14mg		26%
Carbohydrates 86.43g		29%
Dietary Fiber 3.56g		14%
Sugar 49.64g		
Sugar Alcohols 0.00g		
Net Carbohydrates 82.87g		
Protein 29.50g		59%

Lunch

Amount Per Serving		
Calories	360.49	
Calories From Fat (28%)	102.59	
		% Daily Value
Total Fat 11.92g		18%
Saturated Fat 1.53g		8%
Cholesterol 36.12mg		12%
Sodium 156.64mg		7%
Potassium 994.64mg		28%
Carbohydrates 39.53g		13%
Dietary Fiber 10.53g		42%
Sugar 10.64g		
Sugar Alcohols 0.00g		
Net Carbohydrates 29.00g		
Protein 26.49g		53%

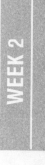

WEEK 2

Dinner

Amount Per Serving		
Calories	641.62	
Calories From Fat (9%)	60.20	
		% Daily Value
Total Fat 7.13g		11%
Saturated Fat 0.98g		5%
Cholesterol 111.25mg		37%
Sodium 849.90mg		35%
Potassium 1533.13mg		44%
Carbohydrates 85.16g		28%
Dietary Fiber 11.07g		44%
Sugar 28.67g		
Sugar Alcohols 0.00g		
Net Carbohydrates 74.09g		
Protein 44.33g		89%

See p. 135 for complete meal.

DAY 15

Breakfast

Amount Per Serving		
Calories	329.47	
Calories From Fat (35%)	116.17	
		% Daily Value
Total Fat 13.11g		**20%**
Saturated Fat 2.73g		**14%**
Cholesterol 8.72mg		**3%**
Sodium 771.31mg		**32%**
Potassium 1558.50mg		**45%**
Carbohydrates 28.85g		**10%**
Dietary Fiber 3.95g		**16%**
Sugar 12.65g		
Sugar Alcohols 0.00g		
Net Carbohydrates 24.90g		
Protein 24.56g		**49%**

Lunch

Amount Per Serving		
Calories	435.96	
Calories From Fat (31%)	136.50	
		% Daily Value
Total Fat 15.90g		**24%**
Saturated Fat 1.68g		**8%**
Cholesterol 18.81mg		**6%**
Sodium 511.31mg		**21%**
Potassium 1104.26mg		**32%**
Carbohydrates 54.77g		**18%**
Dietary Fiber 16.94g		**68%**
Sugar 3.03g		
Sugar Alcohols 0.00g		
Net Carbohydrates 37.83g		
Protein 24.28g		**49%**

Dinner

Amount Per Serving		
Calories	648.64	
Calories From Fat (33%)	212.61	
		% Daily Value
Total Fat 23.72g		**36%**
Saturated Fat 6.51g		**33%**
Cholesterol 52.66mg		**18%**
Sodium 1268.83mg		**53%**
Potassium 1770.46mg		**51%**
Carbohydrates 52.09g		**17%**
Dietary Fiber 11.62g		**46%**
Sugar 13.04g		
Sugar Alcohols 0.00g		
Net Carbohydrates 40.47g		
Protein 52.21g		**104%**

Evening Snack

Amount Per Serving		
Calories	73.82	
Calories From Fat (4%)	2.88	
		% Daily Value
Total Fat 0.35g		**1%**
Saturated Fat 0.04g		**0%**
Cholesterol 0.00mg		**0%**
Sodium 1.35mg		**0%**
Potassium 122.70mg		**4%**
Carbohydrates 19.14g		**6%**
Dietary Fiber 3.24g		**13%**
Sugar 13.71g		
Sugar Alcohols 0.00g		
Net Carbohydrates 15.90g		
Protein 0.70g		**1%**

WEEK 3

See p. 136 for complete meal.

DAY 16

Breakfast

Amount Per Serving		
Calories	393.92	
Calories From Fat (22%)	87.76	
		% Daily Value
Total Fat 10.52g		**16%**
Saturated Fat 2.01g		**10%**
Cholesterol 9.15mg		**3%**
Sodium 336.32mg		**14%**
Potassium 855.71mg		**24%**
Carbohydrates 68.92g		**23%**
Dietary Fiber 8.38g		**34%**
Sugar 34.10g		
Sugar Alcohols 0.00g		
Net Carbohydrates 60.54g		
Protein 12.93g		**26%**

Lunch

Amount Per Serving		
Calories	476.26	
Calories From Fat (25%)	120.66	
		% Daily Value
Total Fat 13.43g		**21%**
Saturated Fat 5.85g		**29%**
Cholesterol 56.02mg		**19%**
Sodium 530.91mg		**22%**
Potassium 1040.40mg		**30%**
Carbohydrates 53.64g		**18%**
Dietary Fiber 8.03g		**32%**
Sugar 15.91g		
Sugar Alcohols 0.00g		
Net Carbohydrates 45.61g		
Protein 38.75g		**78%**

Dinner

Amount Per Serving		
Calories	566.28	
Calories From Fat (46%)	258.31	
		% Daily Value
Total Fat 29.42g		**45%**
Saturated Fat 3.47g		**17%**
Cholesterol 47.85mg		**16%**
Sodium 586.85mg		**24%**
Potassium 971.80mg		**28%**
Carbohydrates 47.64g		**16%**
Dietary Fiber 13.23g		**53%**
Sugar 7.32g		
Sugar Alcohols 0.00g		
Net Carbohydrates 34.41g		
Protein 30.87g		**62%**

Evening Snack

Amount Per Serving		
Calories	100.00	
Calories From Fat (0%)	0.00	
		% Daily Value
Total Fat 0.00g		**0%**
Saturated Fat 0.00g		**0%**
Cholesterol 7.00mg		**2%**
Sodium 70.00mg		**3%**
Potassium 220.00mg		**6%**
Carbohydrates 21.00g		**7%**
Dietary Fiber 0.00g		**0%**
Sugar 19.00g		
Sugar Alcohols 0.00g		
Net Carbohydrates 21.00g		
Protein 4.00g		**8%**

WEEK 3

See p. 137 for complete meal.

DAY 17

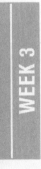

Breakfast

Amount Per Serving		
Calories		370.99
Calories From Fat (13%)		46.60
		% Daily Value
Total Fat 5.63g		**9%**
Saturated Fat 0.46g		**2%**
Cholesterol 0.00mg		**0%**
Sodium 473.82mg		**20%**
Potassium 856.93mg		**24%**
Carbohydrates 76.08g		**25%**
Dietary Fiber 10.96g		**44%**
Sugar 12.27g		
Sugar Alcohols 0.00g		
Net Carbohydrates 65.12g		
Protein 10.27g		**21%**

Lunch

Amount Per Serving		
Calories		323.44
Calories From Fat (54%)		173.31
		% Daily Value
Total Fat 20.32g		**31%**
Saturated Fat 2.73g		**14%**
Cholesterol 46.75mg		**16%**
Sodium 282.19mg		**12%**
Potassium 1321.84mg		**38%**
Carbohydrates 17.92g		**6%**
Dietary Fiber 9.53g		**38%**
Sugar 4.40g		
Sugar Alcohols 0.00g		
Net Carbohydrates 8.39g		
Protein 21.53g		**43%**

Dinner

Amount Per Serving		
Calories		567.97
Calories From Fat (20%)		111.41
		% Daily Value
Total Fat 12.80g		**20%**
Saturated Fat 1.58g		**8%**
Cholesterol 111.25mg		**37%**
Sodium 1144.58mg		**48%**
Potassium 3369.39mg		**96%**
Carbohydrates 76.74g		**26%**
Dietary Fiber 41.31g		**165%**
Sugar 29.18g		
Sugar Alcohols 0.00g		
Net Carbohydrates 35.42g		
Protein 44.71g		**89%**

Evening Snack

Amount Per Serving		
Calories		238.13
Calories From Fat (59%)		141.39
		% Daily Value
Total Fat 16.09g		**25%**
Saturated Fat 10.21g		**51%**
Cholesterol 62.73mg		**21%**
Sodium 103.78mg		**4%**
Potassium 159.19mg		**5%**
Carbohydrates 9.23g		**3%**
Dietary Fiber 0.89g		**4%**
Sugar 4.15g		
Sugar Alcohols 0.00g		
Net Carbohydrates 8.35g		
Protein 14.12g		**28%**

WEEK 3

See p. 138 for complete meal.

DAY 18

Breakfast

Amount Per Serving	
Calories	479.71
Calories From Fat (12%)	56.83
	% Daily Value
Total Fat 6.46g	**10%**
Saturated Fat 0.89g	**4%**
Cholesterol 2.27mg	**1%**
Sodium 936.88mg	**39%**
Potassium 821.78mg	**23%**
Carbohydrates 80.51g	**27%**
Dietary Fiber 4.42g	**18%**
Sugar 37.29g	
Sugar Alcohols 0.00g	
Net Carbohydrates 76.09g	
Protein 26.66g	**53%**

Lunch

Amount Per Serving	
Calories	540.73
Calories From Fat (41%)	221.45
	% Daily Value
Total Fat 26.08g	**40%**
Saturated Fat 3.01g	**15%**
Cholesterol 36.12mg	**12%**
Sodium 546.14mg	**23%**
Potassium 1626.72mg	**46%**
Carbohydrates 51.18g	**17%**
Dietary Fiber 10.57g	**42%**
Sugar 14.89g	
Sugar Alcohols 0.00g	
Net Carbohydrates 40.62g	
Protein 32.08g	**64%**

Dinner

Amount Per Serving	
Calories	493.36
Calories From Fat (42%)	206.12
	% Daily Value
Total Fat 23.00g	**35%**
Saturated Fat 9.43g	**47%**
Cholesterol 66.00mg	**22%**
Sodium 155.63mg	**6%**
Potassium 1254.79mg	**36%**
Carbohydrates 45.28g	**15%**
Dietary Fiber 7.98g	**32%**
Sugar 15.07g	
Sugar Alcohols 0.00g	
Net Carbohydrates 37.31g	
Protein 26.47g	**53%**

Evening Snack

Amount Per Serving	
Calories	83.41
Calories From Fat (5%)	4.49
	% Daily Value
Total Fat 0.54g	**1%**
Saturated Fat 0.03g	**0%**
Cholesterol 0.00mg	**0%**
Sodium 0.37mg	**0%**
Potassium 319.81mg	**9%**
Carbohydrates 20.20g	**7%**
Dietary Fiber 3.91g	**16%**
Sugar 16.53g	
Sugar Alcohols 0.00g	
Net Carbohydrates 16.30g	
Protein 1.78g	**4%**

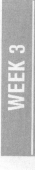

WEEK 3

See p. 139 for complete meal.

DAY 19

Breakfast

Amount Per Serving		
Calories	604.72	
Calories From Fat (14%)	87.57	
		% Daily Value
Total Fat 10.54g		**16%**
Saturated Fat 1.84g		**9%**
Cholesterol 4.92mg		**2%**
Sodium 168.39mg		**7%**
Potassium 2028.12mg		**58%**
Carbohydrates 123.32g		**41%**
Dietary Fiber 12.76g		**51%**
Sugar 80.55g		
Sugar Alcohols 0.00g		
Net Carbohydrates 110.57g		
Protein 16.98g		**34%**

Lunch

Amount Per Serving		
Calories	387.47	
Calories From Fat (55%)	211.63	
		% Daily Value
Total Fat 24.49g		**38%**
Saturated Fat 7.12g		**36%**
Cholesterol 20.41mg		**7%**
Sodium 493.09mg		**21%**
Potassium 1059.26mg		**30%**
Carbohydrates 34.52g		**12%**
Dietary Fiber 12.33g		**49%**
Sugar 5.76g		
Sugar Alcohols 0.00g		
Net Carbohydrates 22.19g		
Protein 13.64g		**27%**

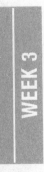

Dinner

Amount Per Serving		
Calories	549.67	
Calories From Fat (16%)	87.21	
		% Daily Value
Total Fat 9.97g		**15%**
Saturated Fat 1.40g		**7%**
Cholesterol 258.55mg		**86%**
Sodium 520.34mg		**22%**
Potassium 1105.71mg		**32%**
Carbohydrates 67.38g		**22%**
Dietary Fiber 14.40g		**58%**
Sugar 5.18g		
Sugar Alcohols 0.00g		
Net Carbohydrates 52.98g		
Protein 49.78g		**100%**

Evening Snack

Amount Per Serving		
Calories	210.04	
Calories From Fat (45%)	94.47	
		% Daily Value
Total Fat 10.84g		**17%**
Saturated Fat 3.97g		**20%**
Cholesterol 5.50mg		**2%**
Sodium 60.46mg		**3%**
Potassium 79.51mg		**2%**
Carbohydrates 26.95g		**9%**
Dietary Fiber 6.00g		**24%**
Sugar 18.30g		
Sugar Alcohols 0.00g		
Net Carbohydrates 20.95g		
Protein 4.51g		**9%**

See p. 140 for complete meal.

DAY 20

Breakfast

Amount Per Serving		
Calories	421.38	
Calories From Fat (10%)	43.48	
		% Daily Value
Total Fat 5.00g		**8%**
Saturated Fat 0.86g		**4%**
Cholesterol 0.63mg		**0%**
Sodium 592.30mg		**25%**
Potassium 945.71mg		**27%**
Carbohydrates 80.80g		**27%**
Dietary Fiber 6.43g		**26%**
Sugar 40.67g		
Sugar Alcohols 0.00g		
Net Carbohydrates 74.37g		
Protein 17.46g		**35%**

Lunch

Amount Per Serving		
Calories	418.44	
Calories From Fat (22%)	93.40	
		% Daily Value
Total Fat 10.83g		**17%**
Saturated Fat 1.57g		**8%**
Cholesterol 36.12mg		**12%**
Sodium 68.15mg		**3%**
Potassium 938.41mg		**27%**
Carbohydrates 59.90g		**20%**
Dietary Fiber 10.69g		**43%**
Sugar 26.55g		
Sugar Alcohols 0.00g		
Net Carbohydrates 49.21g		
Protein 25.42g		**51%**

Dinner

Amount Per Serving		
Calories	734.45	
Calories From Fat (56%)	411.45	
		% Daily Value
Total Fat 48.06g		**74%**
Saturated Fat 6.74g		**34%**
Cholesterol 70.10mg		**23%**
Sodium 169.99mg		**7%**
Potassium 1250.38mg		**36%**
Carbohydrates 51.12g		**17%**
Dietary Fiber 10.35g		**41%**
Sugar 5.32g		
Sugar Alcohols 0.00g		
Net Carbohydrates 40.77g		
Protein 33.62g		**67%**

WEEK 3

See p. 141 for complete meal.

DAY 21

Breakfast

Amount Per Serving		
Calories	352.13	
Calories From Fat (41%)	142.92	
		% Daily Value
Total Fat 16.18g		25%
Saturated Fat 4.29g		21%
Cholesterol 12.01mg		4%
Sodium 831.23mg		35%
Potassium 1296.65mg		37%
Carbohydrates 30.11g		10%
Dietary Fiber 5.49g		22%
Sugar 12.24g		
Sugar Alcohols 0.00g		
Net Carbohydrates 24.62g		
Protein 21.98g		44%

Lunch

Amount Per Serving		
Calories	422.59	
Calories From Fat (41%)	174.52	
		% Daily Value
Total Fat 20.02g		31%
Saturated Fat 2.08g		10%
Cholesterol 89.43mg		30%
Sodium 302.44mg		13%
Potassium 1737.31mg		50%
Carbohydrates 44.93g		15%
Dietary Fiber 8.85g		35%
Sugar 27.07g		
Sugar Alcohols 0.00g		
Net Carbohydrates 36.08g		
Protein 20.76g		42%

Dinner

Amount Per Serving		
Calories	628.49	
Calories From Fat (13%)	78.90	
		% Daily Value
Total Fat 9.25g		14%
Saturated Fat 1.63g		8%
Cholesterol 73.55mg		25%
Sodium 886.26mg		37%
Potassium 1356.85mg		39%
Carbohydrates 79.09g		26%
Dietary Fiber 38.42g		154%
Sugar 17.46g		
Sugar Alcohols 0.00g		
Net Carbohydrates 40.67g		
Protein 41.30g		83%

Evening Snack

Amount Per Serving		
Calories	127.28	
Calories From Fat (65%)	82.71	
		% Daily Value
Total Fat 8.66g		13%
Saturated Fat 5.01g		25%
Cholesterol 1.00mg		0%
Sodium 10.54mg		0%
Potassium 82.62mg		2%
Carbohydrates 10.65g		4%
Dietary Fiber 2.08g		8%
Sugar 8.14g		
Sugar Alcohols 0.00g		
Net Carbohydrates 8.57g		
Protein 0.36g		1%

WEEK 3

See p. 142 for complete meal.

DAY 22

Breakfast

Amount Per Serving		
Calories	241.70	
Calories From Fat (19%)	46.08	
		% Daily Value
Total Fat 5.23g		8%
Saturated Fat 0.54g		3%
Cholesterol 0.00mg		0%
Sodium 1008.01mg		42%
Potassium 1438.31mg		41%
Carbohydrates 31.48g		10%
Dietary Fiber 5.02g		20%
Sugar 22.82g		
Sugar Alcohols 0.00g		
Net Carbohydrates 26.45g		
Protein 18.81g		38%

Lunch

Amount Per Serving		
Calories	604.82	
Calories From Fat (35%)	214.66	
		% Daily Value
Total Fat 24.82g		38%
Saturated Fat 2.31g		12%
Cholesterol 0.00mg		0%
Sodium 1084.30mg		45%
Potassium 1666.66mg		48%
Carbohydrates 86.88g		29%
Dietary Fiber 17.07g		68%
Sugar 20.93g		
Sugar Alcohols 0.00g		
Net Carbohydrates 69.81g		
Protein 16.80g		34%

Dinner

Amount Per Serving		
Calories	695.71	
Calories From Fat (34%)	235.33	
		% Daily Value
Total Fat 26.90g		41%
Saturated Fat 3.15g		16%
Cholesterol 114.71mg		38%
Sodium 587.10mg		24%
Potassium 1332.03mg		38%
Carbohydrates 73.33g		24%
Dietary Fiber 8.82g		35%
Sugar 9.38g		
Sugar Alcohols 0.00g		
Net Carbohydrates 64.51g		
Protein 41.62g		83%

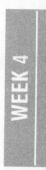

WEEK 4

See p. 143 for complete meal.

DAY 23

Breakfast

Amount Per Serving		
Calories	359.93	
Calories From Fat (21%)	74.18	
		% Daily Value
Total Fat 8.96g		14%
Saturated Fat 0.99g		5%
Cholesterol 2.45mg		1%
Sodium 319.50mg		13%
Potassium 784.55mg		22%
Carbohydrates 65.73g		22%
Dietary Fiber 8.38g		34%
Sugar 30.82g		
Sugar Alcohols 0.00g		
Net Carbohydrates 57.35g		
Protein 10.94g		22%

Lunch

Amount Per Serving		
Calories	443.45	
Calories From Fat (53%)	236.28	
		% Daily Value
Total Fat 27.56g		42%
Saturated Fat 3.28g		16%
Cholesterol 89.43mg		30%
Sodium 270.58mg		11%
Potassium 1288.02mg		37%
Carbohydrates 35.23g		12%
Dietary Fiber 10.37g		41%
Sugar 18.40g		
Sugar Alcohols 0.00g		
Net Carbohydrates 24.86g		
Protein 18.92g		38%

Dinner

Amount Per Serving		
Calories	684.64	
Calories From Fat (28%)	189.31	
		% Daily Value
Total Fat 21.66g		33%
Saturated Fat 5.99g		30%
Cholesterol 50.12mg		17%
Sodium 804.89mg		34%
Potassium 2998.54mg		86%
Carbohydrates 88.15g		29%
Dietary Fiber 5.38g		22%
Sugar 6.43g		
Sugar Alcohols 0.00g		
Net Carbohydrates 82.77g		
Protein 43.36g		87%

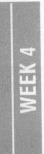

WEEK 4

See p. 144 for complete meal.

DAY 24

Breakfast

Amount Per Serving		
Calories	456.45	
Calories From Fat (18%)	79.96	
		% Daily Value
Total Fat 9.31g		**14%**
Saturated Fat 2.90g		**15%**
Cholesterol 14.94mg		**5%**
Sodium 185.59mg		**8%**
Potassium 724.13mg		**21%**
Carbohydrates 77.42g		**26%**
Dietary Fiber 8.38g		**34%**
Sugar 0.59g		
Sugar Alcohols 0.00g		
Net Carbohydrates 69.04g		
Protein 20.87g		**42%**

Lunch

Amount Per Serving		
Calories	517.84	
Calories From Fat (24%)	121.75	
		% Daily Value
Total Fat 13.56g		**21%**
Saturated Fat 5.91g		**30%**
Cholesterol 56.02mg		**19%**
Sodium 1017.83mg		**42%**
Potassium 1960.59mg		**56%**
Carbohydrates 61.53g		**21%**
Dietary Fiber 8.55g		**34%**
Sugar 25.92g		
Sugar Alcohols 0.00g		
Net Carbohydrates 52.98g		
Protein 40.97g		**82%**

Dinner

Amount Per Serving		
Calories	550.07	
Calories From Fat (36%)	199.16	
		% Daily Value
Total Fat 23.02g		**35%**
Saturated Fat 3.39g		**17%**
Cholesterol 46.75mg		**16%**
Sodium 552.02mg		**23%**
Potassium 1835.37mg		**52%**
Carbohydrates 62.31g		**21%**
Dietary Fiber 16.89g		**68%**
Sugar 16.70g		
Sugar Alcohols 0.00g		
Net Carbohydrates 45.42g		
Protein 29.65g		**59%**

WEEK 4

See p. 145 for complete meal.

DAY 25

Breakfast

Amount Per Serving		% Daily Value
Calories	352.13	
Calories From Fat (41%)	142.92	
Total Fat 16.18g		**25%**
Saturated Fat 4.29g		**21%**
Cholesterol 12.01mg		**4%**
Sodium 831.23mg		**35%**
Potassium 1296.65mg		**37%**
Carbohydrates 30.11g		**10%**
Dietary Fiber 5.49g		**22%**
Sugar 12.24g		
Sugar Alcohols 0.00g		
Net Carbohydrates 24.62g		
Protein 21.98g		**44%**

Lunch

Amount Per Serving		% Daily Value
Calories	463.06	
Calories From Fat (37%)	171.85	
Total Fat 19.76g		**30%**
Saturated Fat 2.52g		**13%**
Cholesterol 14.84mg		**5%**
Sodium 1091.13mg		**45%**
Potassium 883.22mg		**25%**
Carbohydrates 43.87g		**15%**
Dietary Fiber 33.80g		**135%**
Sugar 3.42g		
Sugar Alcohols 0.00g		
Net Carbohydrates 10.07g		
Protein 30.50g		**61%**

Dinner

Amount Per Serving		% Daily Value
Calories	527.12	
Calories From Fat (21%)	110.33	
Total Fat 12.72g		**20%**
Saturated Fat 1.81g		**9%**
Cholesterol 0.00mg		**0%**
Sodium 678.20mg		**28%**
Potassium 1417.89mg		**41%**
Carbohydrates 90.52g		**30%**
Dietary Fiber 15.67g		**63%**
Sugar 10.74g		
Sugar Alcohols 0.00g		
Net Carbohydrates 74.85g		
Protein 17.15g		**34%**

Evening Snack

Amount Per Serving		% Daily Value
Calories	210.04	
Calories From Fat (45%)	94.47	
Total Fat 10.84g		**17%**
Saturated Fat 3.97g		**20%**
Cholesterol 5.50mg		**2%**
Sodium 60.46mg		**3%**
Potassium 79.51mg		**2%**
Carbohydrates 26.95g		**9%**
Dietary Fiber 6.00g		**24%**
Sugar 18.30g		
Sugar Alcohols 0.00g		
Net Carbohydrates 20.95g		
Protein 4.51g		**9%**

WEEK 4

See p. 146 for complete meal.

DAY 26

Breakfast

Amount Per Serving		
Calories		456.80
Calories From Fat (35%)		157.90
		% Daily Value
Total Fat 18.88g		29%
Saturated Fat 1.68g		8%
Cholesterol 2.45mg		1%
Sodium 591.46mg		25%
Potassium 111 1.44mg		32%
Carbohydrates 62.94g		21%
Dietary Fiber 9.20g		37%
Sugar 17.56g		
Sugar Alcohols 0.00g		
Net Carbohydrates 53.74g		
Protein 13.89g		28%

Lunch

Amount Per Serving		
Calories		590.93
Calories From Fat (40%)		233.92
		% Daily Value
Total Fat 27.79g		43%
Saturated Fat 3.36g		17%
Cholesterol 0.00mg		0%
Sodium 167.11mg		7%
Potassium 1519.27mg		43%
Carbohydrates 87.84g		29%
Dietary Fiber 17.69g		71%
Sugar 43.92g		
Sugar Alcohols 0.00g		
Net Carbohydrates 70.16g		
Protein 10.76g		22%

Dinner

Amount Per Serving		
Calories		456.26
Calories From Fat (43%)		198.20
		% Daily Value
Total Fat 22.53g		35%
Saturated Fat 2.62g		13%
Cholesterol 207.19mg		69%
Sodium 569.43mg		24%
Potassium 1002.50mg		29%
Carbohydrates 31.18g		10%
Dietary Fiber 5.28g		21%
Sugar 7.73g		
Sugar Alcohols 0.00g		
Net Carbohydrates 25.91g		
Protein 28.62g		57%

Evening Snack

Amount Per Serving		
Calories		83.41
Calories From Fat (5%)		4.49
		% Daily Value
Total Fat 0.54g		1%
Saturated Fat 0.03g		0%
Cholesterol 0.00mg		0%
Sodium 0.37mg		0%
Potassium 319.81mg		9%
Carbohydrates 20.20g		7%
Dietary Fiber 3.91g		16%
Sugar 16.53g		
Sugar Alcohols 0.00g		
Net Carbohydrates 16.30g		
Protein 1.78g		4%

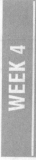

WEEK 4

See p. 147 for complete meal.

DAY 27

Breakfast

Amount Per Serving	
Calories	362.85
Calories From Fat (46%)	166.22
	% Daily Value
Total Fat 18.83g	**29%**
Saturated Fat 2.62g	**13%**
Cholesterol 4.30mg	**1%**
Sodium 254.61mg	**11%**
Potassium 933.69mg	**27%**
Carbohydrates 31.90g	**11%**
Dietary Fiber 3.70g	**15%**
Sugar 20.39g	
Sugar Alcohols 0.00g	
Net Carbohydrates 28.20g	
Protein 18.88g	**38%**

Lunch

Amount Per Serving	
Calories	321.08
Calories From Fat (35%)	112.55
	% Daily Value
Total Fat 13.23g	**20%**
Saturated Fat 1.80g	**9%**
Cholesterol 172.37mg	**57%**
Sodium 439.35mg	**18%**
Potassium 688.00mg	**20%**
Carbohydrates 25.70g	**9%**
Dietary Fiber 5.25g	**21%**
Sugar 5.33g	
Sugar Alcohols 0.00g	
Net Carbohydrates 20.45g	
Protein 27.60g	**55%**

Dinner

Amount Per Serving	
Calories	771.68
Calories From Fat (40%)	306.94
	% Daily Value
Total Fat 35.47g	**55%**
Saturated Fat 3.55g	**18%**
Cholesterol 70.14mg	**23%**
Sodium 991.07mg	**41%**
Potassium 2317.89mg	**66%**
Carbohydrates 75.56g	**25%**
Dietary Fiber 18.55g	**74%**
Sugar 32.10g	
Sugar Alcohols 0.00g	
Net Carbohydrates 57.01g	
Protein 45.82g	**92%**

WEEK 4

See p. 148 for complete meal.

DAY 28

Breakfast

Amount Per Serving	
Calories	631.33
Calories From Fat (27%)	168.93
	% Daily Value
Total Fat 19.48g	30%
Saturated Fat 1.77g	9%
Cholesterol 0.00mg	0%
Sodium 16.06mg	1%
Potassium 520.45mg	15%
Carbohydrates 109.82g	37%
Dietary Fiber 8.44g	34%
Sugar 46.96g	
Sugar Alcohols 0.00g	
Net Carbohydrates 101.37g	
Protein 10.79g	22%

Lunch

Amount Per Serving	
Calories	280.14
Calories From Fat (25%)	70.58
	% Daily Value
Total Fat 8.03g	12%
Saturated Fat 3.92g	20%
Cholesterol 22.25mg	7%
Sodium 685.75mg	29%
Potassium 384.79mg	11%
Carbohydrates 41.83g	14%
Dietary Fiber 3.54g	14%
Sugar 4.07g	
Sugar Alcohols 0.00g	
Net Carbohydrates 38.29g	
Protein 10.46g	21%

Dinner

Amount Per Serving	
Calories	685.26
Calories From Fat (50%)	344.93
	% Daily Value
Total Fat 38.60g	59%
Saturated Fat 8.44g	42%
Cholesterol 47.75mg	16%
Sodium 412.16mg	17%
Potassium 1719.51mg	49%
Carbohydrates 42.67g	14%
Dietary Fiber 11.61g	46%
Sugar 13.27g	
Sugar Alcohols 0.00g	
Net Carbohydrates 31.06g	
Protein 26.45g	53%

WEEK 4

See p. 149 for complete meal.

APPENDIX B:

SHOPPING LIST FOR THE 28-DAY MEAL PLAN

Baking products
Brown sugar
Honey, strained or extracted
Sugar
Beverages
Red wine
White wine
Bread
Bread crumbs
Corn tortillas
Flour tortillas
English muffins
Whole-wheat bread
Canned seafood
Blue crab
Tuna
Canned vegetables
Artichoke hearts
Canned tomatoes
Chickpeas
Kidney beans
Tomato paste
Tomato sauce
Waterchestnuts, Chinese, canned solids
and liquids

Condiments
Dijon mustard
Horseradish
Soy sauce
Worcestershire sauce
Cooking oils and shortening
Canola oil
Cooking spray
Olive oil
Dairy
2% milk
Cream cheese
Eggs
Egg substitute, liquid
Feta
Grated parmesan cheese
Low fat yogurt
Sour cream
Unsalted butter
Dried beans and rice
Black beans
Dried fruit
Dried cherries
Dried cranberries

Flours
  Corn starch
Fresh seafood
  Dungeness crab
Frozen vegetables
  Frozen peas
Fruit and vegetable juices
  Lemon juice
Meat and poultry
  Beef top sirloin
  Chicken breast
Nuts and seeds
  Almonds
  Dry roasted almonds
  Pecans
  Sesame seeds
Pasta
  Linguine
Produce
  Apples (tart, peeled or unpeeled)
  Asparagus
  Avocados
  Bananas
  Beets
  Blueberries
  Broccoli florets
  Brown mushrooms
  Cabbage
  Carrots
  Cauliflower
  Celery
  Cilantro
  Cucumber
  Fresh basil
  Fresh oregano
  Fresh sage
  Fresh tarragon
  Garlic
  Ginger root

Grapefruit
Green bell peppers
Green snap beans
Leeks
Lettuce
Lime juice
Mushrooms
Onions
Orange juice
Oranges
Parsley
Peaches
Portabella mushrooms
Red bell peppers
Red onions
Romaine lettuce
Scallions
Seedless raisins
Shallots
Spinach
Tomatoes
Yellow bell peppers
Salad dressings
  Mayonnaise
Sauces and gravies
  Balsamic vinegar
Spices and seasonings
  Basil (ground)
  Bay leaf
  Black pepper
  Cayenne pepper
  Chili powder
  Cinnamon (ground)
  Cumin seed
  Curry powder
  Dried dill weed
  Dry mustard
  Fresh thyme
  Garlic powder

Ginger (ground)

Nutmeg (ground)

Oregano (ground)

Paprika

Pepper

Red pepper flakes

Salt

Tarragon (ground)

Thyme (ground)

Turmeric (ground)

Vanilla extract

Syrups and sauces

Fish sauce

Tabasco sauce

Unknown grocery aisle

(or salad dressing)

Alfalfa seeds, sprouted, raw

Anchovies

Apples and Blackberries

Arrowroot flour

Avocados

Beef, flank, separable lean and fat, trimmed to 0% fat, all grades, raw

Black Cherry Juice

Blackberries

Broccoli

Butternut squash

Camembert

Cantaloupe, fresh

Carrot juice

Cauliflower

Celery, chopped

Cereals ready-to-eat, corn, whole wheat, rolled oats, presweetened, single brand

Cereals, QUAKER Multigrain Oatmeal, dry

Cereals, QUAKER Quick Oats, Dry

Cherry tomatoes

Clam and tomato juice

Cod

Dark Chocolate 70 % Cocoa – Lindt

Fast foods, scallops, breaded and fried

Flaxseed Meal

Flaxseed oil

Frozen green bell peppers

Frozen peas and onions

Frozen sour cherries

Garlic Shrimp Wrap

Granulated sugar (optional)

Hearts of palm, canned

Honeydew, fresh

Ice creams, Breyers, Fat-Free Vanilla Double Churned

Kalamata olives

Kale, raw

Lamb loin

Long grain brown rice

Low fat vanilla yogurt

Macadamia nuts

Mangos

Miso

Mountain yam, Hawaii, raw

Multigrain Cheerios

Nuts, cashew nuts, raw

Panko (Whole Wheat) Bread Crumbs

Papayas, raw

Parmesan cheese topping, fat free

Pearled barley

Peas

Pineapple

Pita bread

Plain bagels

Pomegranate Juice

Radishes

Raspberries

Ricotta

Salmon

Scallops

Seeds, Flaxseed

Shrimp

Smart Balance

Snow peas

Sour red cherries

Stonyfield Farm Vanilla Nonfat Frozen
  Yogurt

Strawberries

Sweet potato

T-bone steak

Tomato and vegetable juice, low
  sodium

Tuna

V–8 Calcium enriched vegetable juice
  (8 oz)

Vegetable Stock

Walnut oil

Walnuts, halves

Walnuts, coarsely chopped

Wheat bran muffins

Whipping cream (optional)

Whole-wheat crackers

Yam

Vinegars

Red wine vinegar

Rice wine vinegar

ACKNOWLEDGMENTS

Arthritis is a multifaceted and challenging subject. To write about it in a way that is both comprehensive and comprehensible has required the help, advice, and encouragement of many people, all of whom played key roles in turning a simple idea into what I hope is a successful book.

Ernie Tremblay, you are a great medical writer. You are able to take complex topics and put them into a language that all patients will understand. It has been a pleasure working with you on this project.

One of the most wonderful aspects of writing a book of this type has been my working with many health professionals who are dedicated to helping patients with arthritis. A special thanks to Dr. Alison Leon for her many contributions, keen insight, and sound advice. Thank you to Sherri Glasser, R.P.T, and Faye Grand, O.T.C., whose years of experience as therapists provided me with their expert guidance during my development of the exercise program. I am grateful to Marguerite Eng, R.D., whose extensive, professional nutritional experience was invaluable in reviewing the recipes and the meal plan.

I would like to especially thank Dee Jae Diliberto for her generous donation of her time. Her good nature and upbeat attitude became a model for all involved with this book.

Thank you to my agent Ed Claflin for so strongly believing in this project and doing such a great job as my representative.

My deepest gratitude to the editors at Da Capo Press, including Marnie Cochran, Marco Pavia, and Matthew Lore, for their careful and inspired editing of the text.

Sharon J., Deborah M., John DeMaro, and Jay Silverman, you have all contributed in very special ways in bring this book to completion.

Thank you to my staff, who for years have dedicated themselves to helping me to provide the finest care to my patients.

A special thank you to my patients, who have shown me that there is no greater honor than being their physician, and that there is no greater satisfaction than helping them down the road to good health.

And finally to Jerry, Harriet, David, and Mary, who started me down this path and showed me the way.

INDEX